LONE 🌲 PINE

# RUNNING
## START TO FINISH

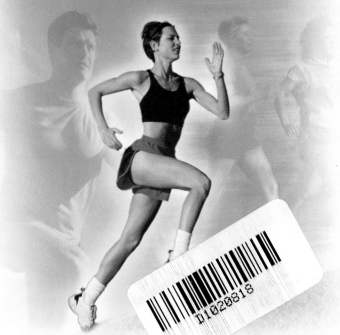

D1020818

# John Stanton

**The Publisher: Lone Pine Publishing**

| | | |
|---|---|---|
| 206, 10426 – 81 Ave. | 202A, 1110 Seymour St. | 1901 Raymond Ave. SW, Suite C |
| Edmonton, AB  T6E 1X5 | Vancouver, BC  V6B 3N3 | Renton, WA  98055 |
| Canada | Canada | USA |

**Website:** http://www.lonepinepublishing.com/

**Canadian Cataloguing in Publication Data**

Stanton, John, 1948-
  Running

ISBN 1-55105-096-X

  1. Running. I. Title.
GV1061.S653 1999            796.42            C99-910049-1

*Editorial Director:* Nancy Foulds
*Project Editor:* Roland Lines
*Production Manager:* David Dodge
*Design & Production:* Michelle Bynoe
*Cover Design:* Rob Weidemann
*Cover Photo Illustration:* David Dodge and Rob Weidemann
*Separations & Film:* Creative Edge Graphic Design

All photographs in this book are provided by John Stanton, Mike O'Dell and Mario Pietramala, except for the following: photos on pp. 96, 167, 169, 242 and 253 are courtesy of the National Capital Marathon; the photo on p. 211 is courtesy of Phil Marsh; the photos on pp. 19, 22, 29, 37, 42, 43, 47, 66, 74, 81, 84, 88, 90, 108, 109, 110, 140, 142, 204, 212, 255, 256 and 258 are courtesy of David Dodge.

We acknowledge the financial support of the Government of Canada through the Book Publishing Industry Development Program (BPIDP) for our publishing activities.

*PC:* 01                                                        Canadä

# Contents

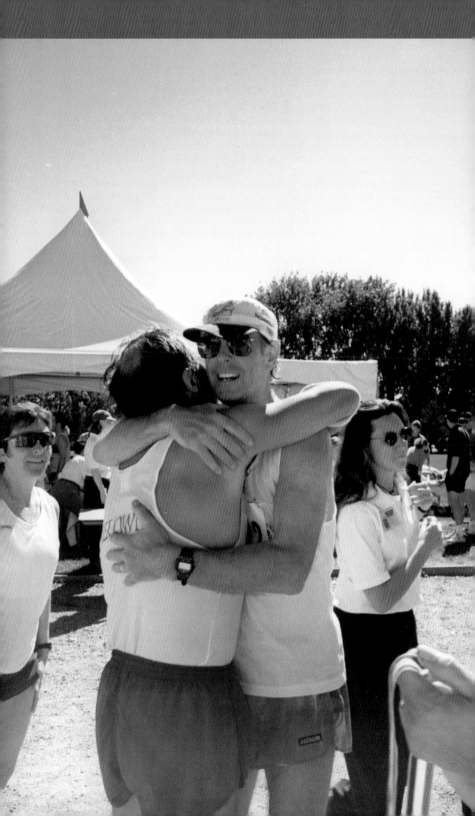

# Preface

Every day, more and more pressure is put on the individual to be accountable for his or her own health and well-being. This book is for those folks who want to take control of their lives and enjoy the resulting improvements in their quality of life. I was an overweight, out-of-shape, chain-smoking corporate executive who took up running to lose weight. Not only did I lose the weight and quit smoking, I experienced the benefits of a lifestyle change by substituting positive addictions for negative ones.

I wrote this book to share some of the knowledge I have gained about the great sport of running over the past 15 years. Running, the simple act of putting one foot in front of the other, has evolved into a whole complex sport. This book deals with the many issues and tips that will allow you to enjoy running for the sheer joy of good health—it is intended to add value to the quality of life you now enjoy.

Running, like most things in life, is not about individual performance but rather about teamwork. Writing a book brings this message close to home. So, to my family, our Running Room family, our extended family of runners and the great folks at Lone Pine, I say thank you for the contribution. Each of you significantly improved the quality of the content. I thank you all.

Specifically, I want to thank Melissa Stanton and Dr. Harvey Sternberg for their considerable technical contribution and Linda Caldwell for her editorial assistance, as well as Cary Moretti, Trevor Shapcot, Tara Hafso, Mike Mendzat, Mike O'Dell, Jason Stanton and my wife, Bev.

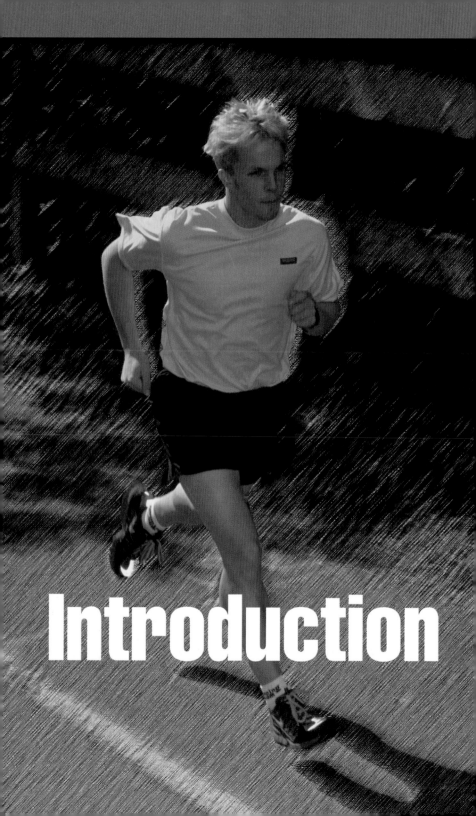

# Introduction

Studies continue to show that exercise yields an enriched lifestyle. At one time, we thought that running might not add years to one's life but it would certainly add quality. Recently, however, we have learned that not only will runners enjoy a better quality of life, they will in fact live longer—up to six years longer if they exercise regularly.

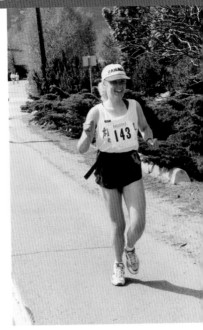

If you are like many folks today, looking for a fitness program that fits into your busy lifestyle, running may be the optimum workout for you. Running burns fat at a high rate, relieves stress, improves your self-esteem and helps you sleep better. It also improves your energy levels, endurance, strength and muscle definition, increases your odds against heart diseases, improves your cardiovascular system and helps you relax. Running can help depression, give you a positive attitude in everything you do, raise your metabolic rate, polish up your self-image, awaken your sex life and give you that "I feel good" feeling about yourself and your whole life. You will work, play and sleep with an improved attitude towards life—not a bad payback for an investment of 30 to 40 minutes, five days a week, to do something we once called play.

## "Why Run?"

**Rewards of improved fitness:**

- **improved self-esteem**

- **stress relief**

- **healthier eating habits.**

**The improved self-esteem will come quickly as you exercise. You will find yourself more positive and more productive at work and at play. You will also have more energy and you will generally start to enjoy life more. As your energy and outlook improve, the people you live and work with will start to enjoy your company more.**

# The New Running Boom

As we enter the new millennium, we are also entering a new running boom. The seventies and eighties saw the first running boom as Baby Boomers with type-A personalities got themselves into fitness—they took up running and squash—to pit their competitive juices against each other. They played to win the game. The new running boom sees people running and winning the game of health and fitness through participation, not competition. We run for weight control, stress relief and that positive feeling that exercise gives as a reward for our efforts. Much has been written about the loneliness of the long-distance runner, but as we learned to train in groups, we learned just how social running can be.

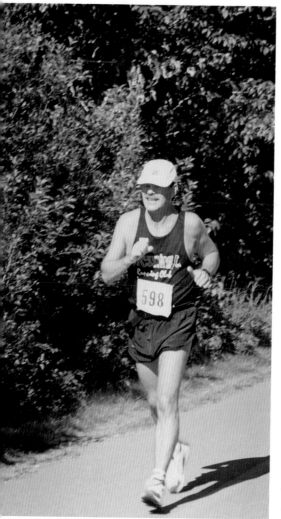

Running has changed from being an exclusively competitive sport to a lifestyle workout that can be done for years and can add years to your life. Listen to the youth of today as they discuss their daily routine: they refer to going for their daily workout much as their parents referred to brushing their teeth or combing their hair. Fitness has become a way of life. A workout can be a run, a swim, a fitness class, a squash game—the difference is that they get in a daily workout without being as obsessive and compulsive as the folks of the seventies and eighties. They appreciate the balance that a varied workout gives them.

We have reached new levels in performance by using the lessons of the first running boom to modify some of our former training programs. Many folks who jumped into running during the first boom soon dropped out because they did too much, too fast, too soon and for too long. The primary difference today is a decrease in the intensity of the workout, which has made the sport achievable and enjoyable to many folks who once thought they could not call themselves runners—never mind athletes—except on the odd occasion. We have learned a great deal in the past few years about how to get the optimum performance out of a reasonable investment of time and energy, and we have learned some valuable lessons from sports medicine experts about the importance of rest. The equipment available to runners has also improved substantially, and we have learned much about how components like nutrition can affect our performance, both as athletes and in life.

One of the key indicators that people run for different reasons today than they did in the early eighties is race distances. The fastest-growing race distance in North America today is the 5-K. This "fun" distance is one that runners of all ages and fitness levels can accept as a reasonable challenge. It also is a distance that attracts people who simply enjoy the camaraderie of a run and the muffins and goodies in the food tent. Many events are now called "fun runs," where most were once called "races."

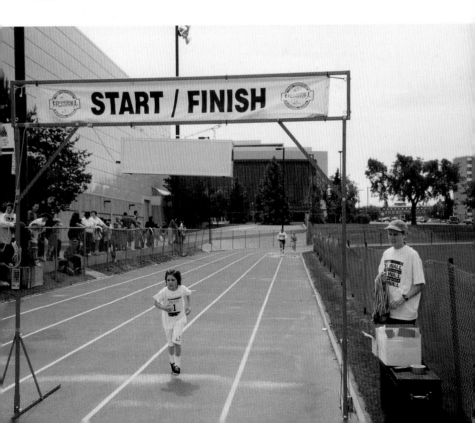

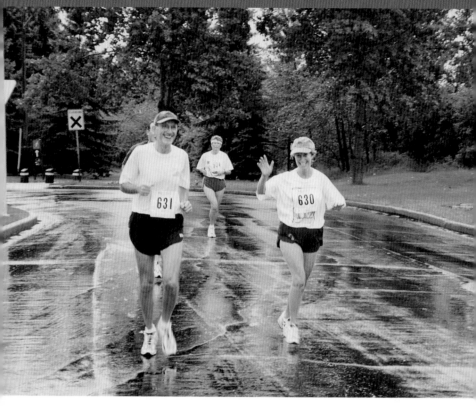

The changing attitude towards the competitive side of running has not been limited to the 5-K and 10-K distances; it has changed right up to the marathon distance, that mythical, magical distance that many people find to be the ultimate test—the test of ordinary folks doing the extraordinary. Marathons continue to grow in participation, and the mean finishing time continues to increase. In the early eighties, many marathons had mean finishing times just over 3 hours. I recall being at one marathon where at the 4-hour mark the race officials came out and asked anyone still on the course to move to the sidewalk. They also took the runners' numbers. The only people at the finish line for those left on the course were their families and friends. Well, much has changed since then; most major marathons today have mean finishing times that exceed 4 hours.

Runners are the free spirits of the new running boom. As you let yourself experience the benefits of a regular exercise program, you will discover that running is actually fun! Today, we have learned that an athlete is waiting in all of us.

# Motivation, Inspiration, Belief in Yourself

*Where do you find the motivation?* Non-runners will often ask you this question, along with, *How many miles in a marathon? Did you win?* and, if you didn't, *Why not?* You will even occasionally ask yourself, *Why the heck am I doing this?*

As you run, you will soon develop your own reasons for running. Some of us run for physical health; lots of us run for weight control; some run for stress release; some run to socialize. Most of us run to feel good about ourselves and for the general well-being we feel after a run. These motivating forces are what generally keep you running when the negative side of your brain tries to convince you to skip a run.

We all know that feeling of coming home tired from a hard day at work or school, thinking, *I can't run tonight. I'm too tired!* A test I give myself is to agree to change into my running gear and run for 10 minutes. At the end of 10 minutes, if I'm still tired I can return home. Fatigue at that point of the run is likely a sign that you are overtraining, dehydrated, hungry or truly tired, so turn back.

Rest is part of every good training program, and if you need it, for whatever reason, then take the rest. One short day or rest day will often enable you to come back to your running the next day with a renewed vigour. For the most

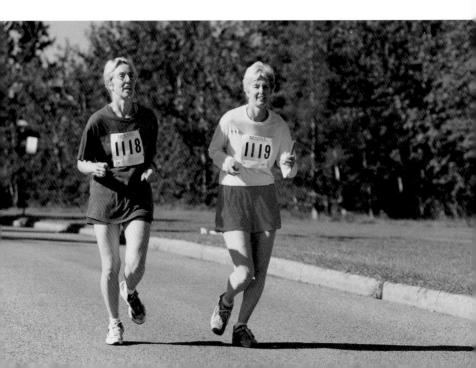

part, however, by the time 10 minutes comes around I have forgotten that I was tired—I'm usually enjoying my run to the point that I don't remember to check the time.

There are no short cuts to fitness, but what runners have learned in the last few years is to keep it fun. The first running boom used hard, intense workouts to pump up the fitness folks of the eighties, but today, thanks to another 20 years of training research, we have learned how to "train with a brain" and dump the

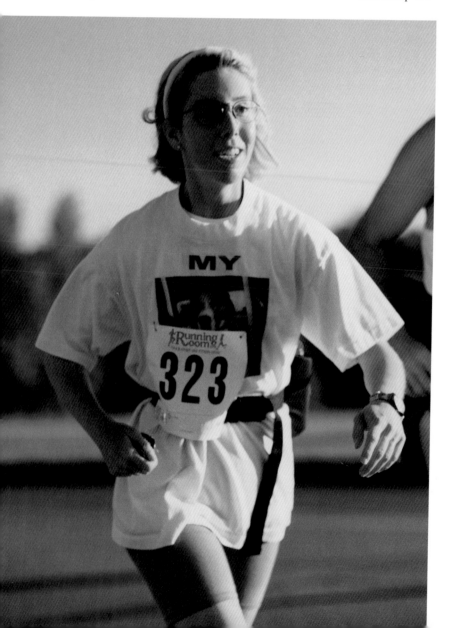

old "no pain, no gain" theory. The improved training techniques have allowed a lot of folks to become runners when 10 years ago neither they nor some of the so-called experts would have thought it was possible. Also, as the intensity of the workout decreases, so does the injury risk. Remember, running is play; it is supposed to be fun.

Do not let your current assessment of your body image be a concern. Running will not only help in your weight loss, it will help your confidence and self-esteem. Running is a great way to take control of your attitude. The sense of accomplishment and well-being that comes from a long run is all the reward most runners look for today. We have discovered that the euphoria that comes from the last 100 metres of a road race can be a powerful motivation in other facets of our lives. We soon learn that that sense of accomplishment breeds an improved self-esteem in just about everything we do. We find we have more energy and feel more positive about the challenges we face in our homes, our work and our communities. Runners care about themselves, and taking control and caring for your own health is a good start towards caring for others.

Do not let anyone tell you that you will never be a runner. Time and time again, I have seen individuals make the decision to take control of their lives and succeed. Anyone who can currently run for 1 minute and walk for 1 minute can, in as little as 10 weeks, run for 20 minutes non-stop. Once you are running for 20 minutes, you will then be well on your way to a lifetime of good health and fitness. You will find that you have more energy, your life will become more enjoyable and those folks that you live with will find you more fun to be around.

## Positive Self Talk

- I am in control of my own life.
- I can achieve any intelligent goal I set for myself.
- I believe in myself and the people around me.
- I treat every day as a new challenge to improve myself in some way.

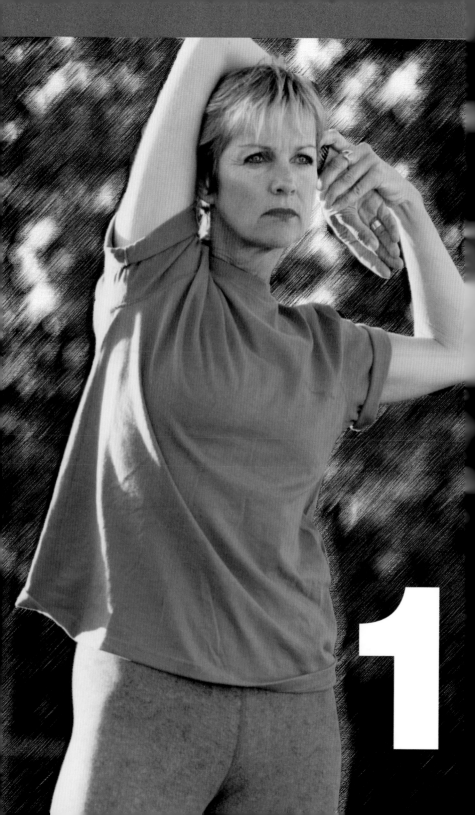

**1**

# Getting Started

Let's talk about designing your training program. One of the first things to consider is that every runner is unique, so your program must be modified according to your individual requirements, talents and commitment. You recognize that your fingerprints are unique, but so are a number of other factors that you should work around your running program: your distinctive physiological characteristics (body type, resting and maximum heart rates and the basic ability of your body to use oxygen); your individual needs (what you want to achieve through exercise); and the different demands placed on you by your commitments to your family, friends, community and work.

## Fitting It All In

All of us are faced with the challenge of fitting a workout into our busy daily schedules. Our friends, families and communities all require time, and in today's marketplace many people have great demands placed on them at work. Our personal time is becoming very precious.

So, just how do we have time to fit it all in? To start with, make a daily appointment with yourself for your own health and fitness. It is not selfish; it is necessary. In order to care about the other people in your life, you must first care about yourself. If not, just how are you going to be any good to them?

One of the more common questions I get asked is, *What is the best time of the day to run?* Well, here are the answers I have received from thousands of runners over the years. As you will see, there is no best time. There is, however, a best time for you.

### I like to get out of bed and run to start my day.

An early morning run works best for some people. It starts their day off and gets them in the right mental shape for the day. They find that they eat less, are more productive throughout the day and then come home to relax without the stress of having to get their run in when they are tired. They also tell me they sleep well at night.

### I like to run at noon; it's the perfect time for me.

Runners that run at noon tell me their run breaks up the day, gives them an attitude change for the afternoon and forces them to eat a light lunch.

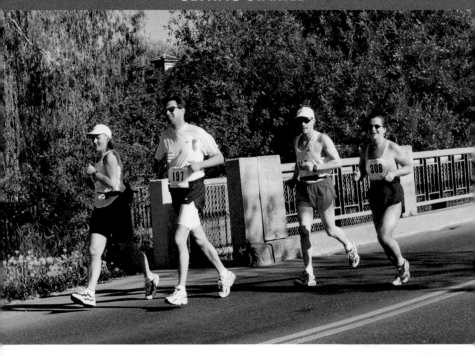

## I like to run right after work, before supper.

These runners say they can come home from work tired mentally, but then go out for a run and come back feeling rejuvenated. They say that the run after work and before supper makes them enjoy their evenings more, and for many of them exercise is an appetite suppressant.

## I like to run before I go to sleep.

Some runners tell me that the late evening run is grand. It relaxes them for the night and is a great time to meditate about life's challenges and find the simple solutions that a run can deliver. They also like to brag that the run revs up their metabolism, which continues to burn fat as they sleep. Sounds like a great deal for those of us looking for a fat burning advantage.

So, when is the best time to run? Remember that we are each unique and that running is supposed to be adding value to your life, so find the time of day that fits your individual schedule. (For me, an evening run just makes me a bigger fan of late night television—I return from a late run full of new energy, stay up late and then find myself tired the next day.) Use your runs to improve your mental as well as your physical well-being. Keep your running time as a stress-buster—most of us have enough stress in our lives that we do not need to add any more.

# STOP PROCRASTINATING

- Plan and schedule your daily workouts.

- Be flexible within your schedule. Just commit to completing the workout.

- Be creative in planning your workouts. Use normal down time or waiting time to get in that run, stretch session or cross-training session.

- Read, listen or watch something humorous. A good laugh gets rid of most stress.

- Vary your workouts. Running the same distance or course every day can soon lead to boredom. A little speed or some hill repeats will put some spring back into your stride.

- Run with a buddy. You will motivate each other.

- Imagine yourself in a race leading a pack that is 25 metres behind you. Push just a little.

- In a safe area, put on headphones and listen to some music, a motivational tape or a comedy tape.

- Mix it up: change the time of day you normally run; run in a different direction; run a new work-out; or read up on some new running drills to try.

- Run past a hospital to remind yourself how fortunate you are to have your good health. It is a fragile gift you must look after.

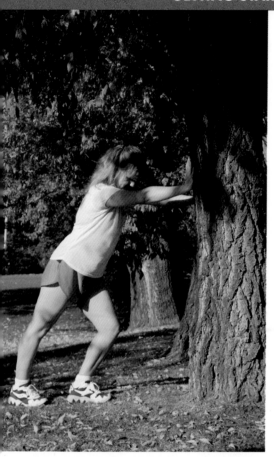

# Goal Setting

To get the most out of your training program, you should set an ultimate goal and then set several smaller goals to get you there. Your ultimate goal might be to run a particular race, but before you run that race you must first train consistently, and it can help to set some smaller, shorter-distance races as targets to test yourself along the way. (Interestingly, many marathon runners will tell you that the true reward comes from the training, not the marathon itself.)

Your goals can be qualitative, or they can be quantitative: a qualitative long-term goal might be to make fitness part of your daily routine, just like brushing your teeth or combing your hair; a quantitative long-term goal might be to run a specific marathon when your birthday takes you into a new decade.

Set short-term goals that allow you to savour some of your training rewards: your first goal might be to run continuously for 20 minutes. One good goal at the start of any program is to run for 30 days without an injury, which will force you to listen to your body.

In your program, you will have five kinds of goals:

1. a daily goal to get out the door every day;

2. a self-acceptance goal—condition yourself to the acceptance that daily fitness is part of your lifestyle;

3. a performance goal for a season—either a distance goal, such as running a 10-K, or a time goal, such as breaking 45 minutes for a 10-K;

4. a dedication goal or a special goal for a season, something that will motivate you to continue training throughout the year—dedicate your

year to the memories of a loved one, or dedicate your goal to proving you can do it when others believe you cannot;

5. a dream goal—a big race or special distance that seems just slightly out of reach but achievable.

If your goals are intelligent and realistic, you will be more likely to succeed and not get discouraged part-way through your training. There is no special formula for where you should start or the rate at which you should progress, but take care not to let your new-found fitness carry you beyond improvement into overuse. Don't look at the people around you, look at where you are now and start a program of improvement from that point. Set a current benchmark and try to improve by approximately 10 percent a week. (Keeping a limit of 10 percent a week allows you to improve while minimizing your risk of injury.)

To help you along the way, in both assessment and encouragement, start a logbook. A daily log will reinforce your progress towards your individual goals— there is a certain pleasure that comes from recording your workouts and assessing the quality of the effort. Record the distance you ran, where you ran and the type of run (e.g., hill workout, long and slow, speed training). Include notes on how you felt, especially if your stress level was above normal, and abnormal weather conditions.

Be sure to monitor and evaluate your training, adjusting your program and goals to your progress and the other facets of your life. Use your logbook to document any changes in your circum- stances and the corresponding adjustments to your short- term and long-term goals. Now, this is not a free-ride ticket that lets you back off your training for every little interference, but you should back off if conditions warrant. For example, if the weather becomes extremely hot, you must intelligently modify the intensity of your training

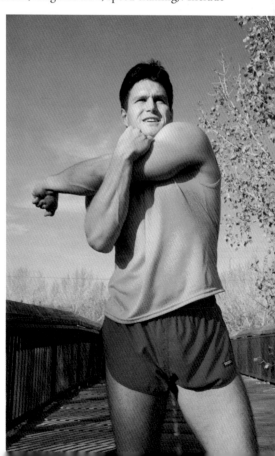

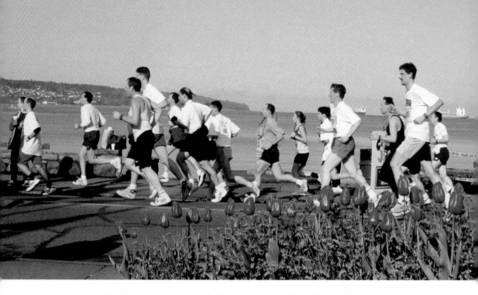

program; or if a busy work schedule leaves you tired, and you have bad runs on two consecutive days, you need to progress more slowly.

Remember that sometimes your daily goal will be to have a rest day. Rest is a good four-letter word that lets your body rebuild and get stronger—sports medicine experts say you need 48 hours to recover from a hard workout—so it should be a scheduled part of every training program.

The setting of athletic goals, the discipline of following a regimented program towards specific goals and the recording of your progress will transfer over into the other parts of your life. Studies continue to prove that people who are physically active are more positive in their approach to challenges, have more energy and eat better. These added benefits and feelings of improved health are some of the reason runners become highly self-motivated over a period of time.

## Join the Top 10 Percent

Only 10 percent of the population in North America, England and Australia do enough exercise to break a sweat.

# Top 10 Reasons People Take Up a Running Program

1. Stress relief.

2. Weight control.

3. Feeling of well-being.

4. To meet people who share similar values of a healthy lifestyle.

5. It's a simple fitness program that can be done anywhere, anytime and with little special equipment.

6. Low cost of equipment.

7. Positive self motivation.

8. Improvement of self-image.

9. Pursuit of a specific race goal.

10. The group's positive peer pressure to stay motivated.

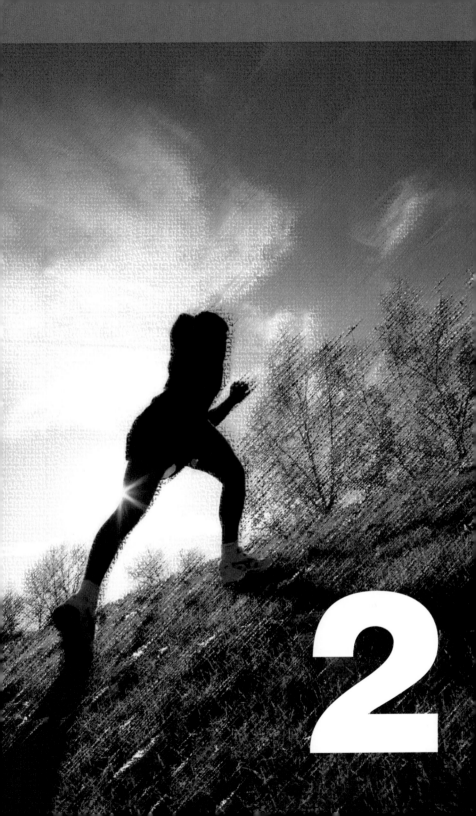

# Building Your Program

## Basic Principles of Training

Now that you know where you want to start and where you want to end up, it is important to implement a program that will ensure success. One way is to apply the basic principles of training—a set of "rules" to follow when you develop your training program, no matter what your starting level.

### The Training Adaptation

Your body will only adapt to unaccustomed stress. In order to stimulate a training response, the stress of a training session must be strong enough to upset the balance of the various functional systems of the body (the cardiovascular system, the skeletal system, the muscular system, etc.). As a result, the body reorganizes the various systems to re-establish a balanced state. This reorganization is the training adaptation, often referred to as supercompensation. The degree of adaptation depends on the degree of imbalance induced: hard training will induce a greater degree of imbalance, and a greater degree of adaptation, than easy training.

### Stress; then Rest

In running, more is not always better. The most common error many runners make is to do too much, too soon. The toughest thing for many athletes to understand is that *rest is part of training*. Rest allows your body to recover and adapt to the stresses of your training program. Stressing yourself without rest will result in poor performance and you will risk an injury. If you do not build rest into your training program, your body will build it in for you through injury.

For a training adaptation to occur, there must be a period of rest after a training session to provide time for regeneration. The amount of time required depends

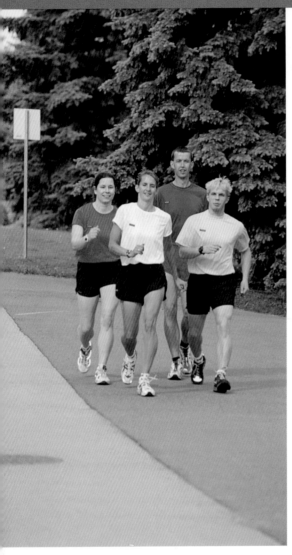

on the degree to which the body's systems were upset. For example, a training session in which you run either faster or longer than usual (or both) will require a longer rest period for regeneration to occur. If the rest period is too short, the body will not have time to adapt before the next training session and the full training effect will not be observed. On the other hand, if the rest period is too long, the training adaptation will start to fade before your next training session.

Observing proper rest periods is where consistency and moderation of training become very important aspects of your program. If you have a bad week and miss some training sessions, don't try and make up for it by adding in those missed sessions during the next week. You will only shorten your regeneration time and hinder the adaptive process.

Training once a week is not too helpful, either, because the rest period is too long and some, if not all, of the training adaptation will fade before the next session.

Complete regeneration is not always necessary between each training session—quite often, runners don't feel fatigued until after several training sessions in which only partial adaptation was able to take place. Don't push it too far; be sure your program allows for at least partial recovery between each training session or week of training.

## Progressive Overload

If you impose the same level of stress (at the same frequency) with each training session, that stress is no longer unaccustomed and no further adaptation will occur. If you want greater training adaptations, your running program should become progressively more difficult through the weeks and months of training.

**CH. 2**

The most common ways to increase your training load are to increase the intensity, frequency or duration of the training sessions. Intensity is how fast you run (or what percentage of your run is uphill); frequency is the number of training sessions in a week; duration is how long each training session lasts.

Be sure to follow the 10 percent rule when you increase your training load: increase your weekly mileage by no more than 10 percent a week. The body needs only slight increases in stress. Too much stress over a short period of time will lead to breakdown rather than training adaptation.

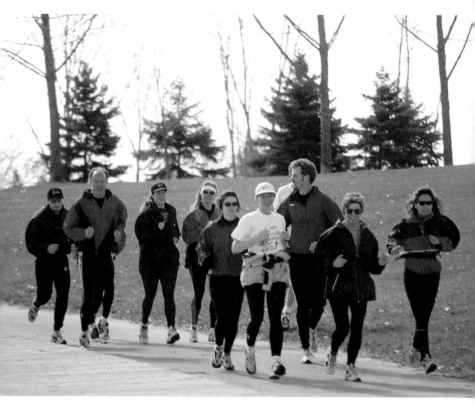

# How Much Rest Do You Need?

**Rest can mean many different things to different people. Getting appropriate rest while you are training doesn't mean inactivity, but if you are planning a training program to improve your 10-K time, playing a five-set tennis match on your rest day won't help, either.**

**Think about what you do during the course of a workday. If your job involves manual labour, you will probably need to be more inactive during your rest time. On the other hand, if you work at a desk for most of the day, total inactivity in your rest time may be unnecessary.**

**Your rested state is also greatly affected by your quality and amount of sleep. Required sleep amounts vary from person to person, but quality is important, too. You may want to ask yourself a few questions when thinking about your sleep quality:**

- **Do you frequently wake up during the night?**

- **Does your job require you to work through the night?**

- **Are you a shift worker? Do you sometimes work days; sometimes nights?**

**People who are frequently interrupted throughout the night or who work nights and sleep during the day need to ensure that they are getting appropriate rest. Poor sleep patterns can adversely affect exercise training and performance.**

## Hard and Easy Days

Hard and easy days are a great addition to a running program. The hard/easy approach to training is based on the theory that gradual increases in training volume or intensity are not as effective as the occasional sharp increase. The hard days are great mental, as well as physical, challenges; the easy days allow for some extra regeneration, even though you're still getting out to exercise. Your hard days shouldn't be so hard that you can't walk for three days afterwards, but they should be hard enough that you need extra rest time. If you are including hard/easy training in your program, be sure you are planning carefully.

CH. 2

# Walk is a Good Four-letter Word

If you're just getting into running, or if you have just begun running longer distances, walking is going to be an integral part of your training sessions. The benefits of walking while run training are not completely understood, but what we do know is that walk breaks provide relief from the aerobic and muscular stresses of running while still providing some exercise stress.

Walk breaks are important for both beginning runners and novice long-distance runners who are attempting to increase their mileage. By incorporating walk breaks into your training program, you can extend the limits of your endurance. For the beginner, walk breaks may make the difference between running for 8 minutes and running for half an hour; walk breaks may allow a novice distance runner to run 20 miles (32 km) rather than 15 miles (24 km).

The walk breaks should be done at a brisk rate to maintain an elevated heart rate and to give the large muscles in your legs a gentle stretch. As you run long distances, your large leg muscles fatigue and your stride begins to shorten; a brisk walk maintains a full range of motion by gently stretching the muscles. The gentle stretch also helps flush the lactic acid that may be building up in the muscles, preventing soreness during the following days.

For the runner who thinks these breaks sound wimpy, call them water breaks. That way, if someone spots you walking just tell them, "I'm not walking I'm on a water break." And it's not all posturing—drinking an adequate amount of water on a regular basis will improve the quality of your training.

It sounds easy, but there are a few rules to follow when you incorporate walk breaks into your training sessions.

- Take walk breaks often (at least one break every 10 minutes).

- Walk briskly and think about increasing your stride during the walk break so you will feel the gentle stretch of your tired muscles.

- Beginner runners need walk breaks more often.

- A walk break is just a break, so be sure it isn't too long. You shouldn't need more than a minute. If a minute is too short, your pace is probably too fast.

- Take walk breaks sooner, rather than later. At the beginning of a run, you are always going to feel better than at the end, but don't wait until you feel fatigued to take your break or it will be too late. Walk breaks used throughout a run delay the onset of fatigue; walk breaks do not restore energy once fatigue has already set in.

- If you don't need walk breaks to complete the distance, don't use them—running is still the best way to increase your fitness. Experienced runners will probably find that they only need to use walk breaks when they run more than 10 miles (16 km).

- Walk breaks enhance your recovery from the long run and give you the edge required to meet the demands of the next high-quality run.

## Base Training

The largest portion (about 50 percent) of your training program should be base training, which prepares your cardiovascular system for future demands and builds your endurance. Base training is especially important for beginning runners, because after a long period of inactivity, your body is not ready for the demands of intense exercise.

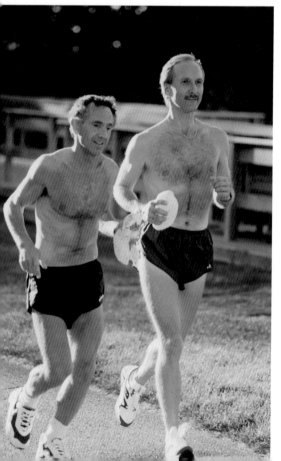

Base training increases the efficiency of the circulatory system by increasing the strength of the heart muscle and by improving blood flow and oxygen delivery to the muscles. The cardiovascular and circulatory systems are the base support systems for all future training. Base training also improves the efficiency of individual muscle fibres, the aerobic energy system and the removal of waste, such as lactic acid, which builds up in muscles during exercise.

For base training to be most effective, volume, rather than intensity, is key. The intensity should elicit a heart rate of between 130 and 150 beats a minute, and it should be maintained for at least 20 to

CH. 2

30 minutes. If you're not quite ready to monitor your heart rate, use the "talk test": while running, you should be able to carry on a conversation with ease and not feel like you are gasping for breath. If you do feel out of breath, slow down.

So, how far should you go? There is an optimum training distance that will allow the body to adapt to its highest aerobic capacity, but it is different for everyone. The physiological returns of running a high weekly distance vary greatly from runner to runner. If you are currently running less than 40 miles (66 km) a week, you have probably not reached your physiological endurance potential; if you are running more than 90 miles (145 km) a week, you are probably going too far; running 60 to 90 miles (96 to 145 km) a week is a physiological gray area. There is a point where increasing your training distance will not elicit any more increases in endurance, and all levels of runners must be careful to avoid the dangers of increasing distances too much or too quickly.

Many people find base training tedious, but the advantage of it is that once you have achieved these training adaptations, they are difficult to lose and easy to maintain.

## Strength Training

Strength is critical to every running event for both men and women, and it should make up 35 percent of your yearly training sessions. Increased strength has a positive effect on both your speed and endurance, because a stronger muscle can work more quickly and has the potential for greater endurance.

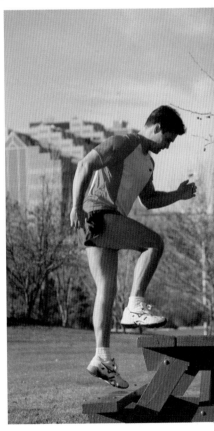

Strength training can be for whole-body strength, as in general conditioning, or for specific strength, which is most effective within the range of motion of a given sport. The most specific method of strength training for running is to overload the leg muscles by running hills or by running faster for short periods of time.

There is a right time and a wrong time to add strength training to your program. Generally, you should not begin strength training until you have developed an adequate base, because the drills required

**CH. 2**

for improved strength will tax your aerobic system as well. If you want, you can improve your overall strength through general body conditioning in a weight room. Runners, however, need to focus on weight workouts that include a full range of motion similar to that used in running. This specific strength training can be part of your general training program. Most runners want strong, supple muscles—they do not want to bulk up—so moderate weights should be used in all exercises. A lightweight workout through a correct range of motion is good for runners. Heavy weights through a limited range of motion can leave the runner tight and fatigued.

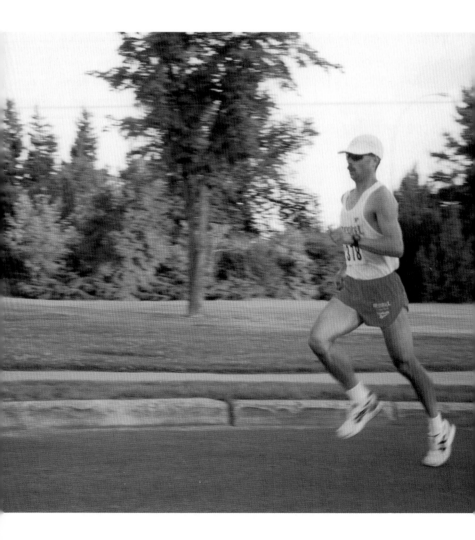

# BUILDING THE HOUSE

## Speed Training

The primary aim of speed work is to strengthen your fitness above your comfort zone. Speed training improves the strength of your running muscles and teaches them the coordination required for faster running.

## Strength Training

Your hill training sessions strengthen the key running muscles in your lower legs, allowing you to shift your weight a bit farther forward on your feet and to use your ankles for efficient mechanical advantage—gaining a stronger push-off. Now you're ready for the fast stuff!

## Base Period

During the base period, you get your cardiovascular system ready to handle future speed demands. Whether you've run before or not, your base period training will improve your cardiovascular efficiency. Your base training can be dramatically improved with slower running or by a combination of running and walking.

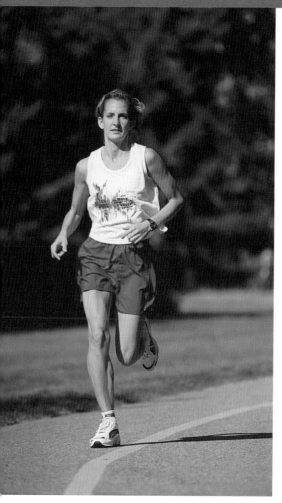

# Speed Training

Nailing on the roof of the house is the last thing we do in our training analogy. Speed training should be thought of as the fine-tuning done in preparation for the race. It should not take place until six to eight weeks before the event, and even then, if you have not completed sufficient base and strength training by this time, speed training may be inappropriate.

The primary purposes of speed training are to teach the body, specifically the running muscles, to function anaerobically, and to train the leg muscles for the strength and coordination they need for faster running. Since speed training is aimed at developing speed, strength and coordination, not endurance, the total distance that you cover during your workout is inconsequential.

Speed training is usually accomplished through interval training. Intervals are fast runs over short distances with a recovery of walking or light running. The distances can vary from 400 meters for the 10-K runner to 1 mile (1.6 km) for the marathon runner. Your interval pace is dependent on your state of conditioning and experience.

Speed training imposes great stresses on the muscular system, so it should only comprise 15 percent of your yearly training plan. Generally, it is done during the fine-tuning stage of your program—adequate endurance and strength are essential before undertaking speed training.

# The Seasonal Approach

To build your program using the seasonal approach, start by dividing the year into three major periods—pre-season, in-season and post-season, for example— to give yourself a general focus for your training program. These divisions should help you organize your program according to which activities are the prerequisites to others. In running, for example, base training is the prerequisite to strength training. The progression through the season generally involves a change from predominantly distance training to strength training to higher-intensity workouts specific to competition later in the season.

## Periodization

If you are currently using the seasonal approach to your training, you are already practising what is known as periodization. Periodization is a way of structuring your training program using a planned program of base training, strength training, speed training, racing and rest to produce a desired performance without becoming overtrained or injured. This approach to training doesn't mean you have to race, but by planning for races it lets you structure your program around the time you would like to be in top shape.

Further dividing your training season into smaller, one-month units will allow you to structure a progressive increase in training while incorporating appropriate rest to allow for regeneration and adaptation. Each one-month training unit should generally focus on one part of the training period. For instance, at the beginning of the training year you may have four or five month-long units where you focus on base training.

The one-month training units each divide into four one-week units. The first two weeks of each month are characterized by developmental training—lower intensity training sessions that focus on building volume. The third week may be highly intensive: it contains considerable volume and requires you to perform at a higher intensity. (It is during the intensive week that most of the training adaptation occurs.) The last week is rehabilitative: it consists of more rest days, and all the training sessions are of a lower intensity and volume. This system of adjusting your training volume and intensity throughout the month will allow you to train through short-term fatigue. You will avoid chronic fatigue, because the week of intensive training is always followed by a recovery week.

Your weekly training program is how you integrate running into the reality of life. The training you include in your weekly schedule will depend on the training season. In the pre-season, for example, when base training is commonly the focus, you won't have to worry about scheduling hill workouts or speed training.

If you train more than four times a week, it is unlikely that you can recover fully between each training session. Careful planning is needed, because you will become more and more fatigued as the week progresses, and the effectiveness of certain types of training will decrease. For technique and speed training to be optimally effective, for example, the runner has to be well rested, so they should be done early in the week. Anaerobic endurance works well in the middle of the week; muscular and aerobic endurance at the end. As a general rule of thumb, the most intense types of training should be scheduled at the beginning of the week. As the week progresses, the intensity should decrease, ending with rest and recovery.

## Low Intensity, High Stress

**Long runs that last more than 90 minutes are considered highly stressful, even if their intensity is light. They should be performed early in the week and definitely during a high-intensity week of training.**

# Training Plateaus

Performance and fitness level are the measures by which we gauge the success or failure of our fitness programs. What most people forget is that as you become more fit, performance and fitness gains require much more work. For an elite runner, for example, many years of hard training may only improve performance by a few minutes ... even seconds.

Even if you're just starting out, you will probably experience plateaus in your training. Improvements in fitness and performance take place almost in a stepwise fashion: increases in fitness are followed by fitness plateaus. The first several steps are high and narrow—the plateaus are short—but as your training continues, the steps become shorter and wider, until you finally reach your fitness ceiling. Near the top of the stairs, where only small gains are made with training, the athlete must pay very close attention to the training loads and rest.

Currently, there is no way to predict your maximum potential, so you'll just have to keep trying to reach higher performance and fitness levels until someone finds a way to measure your potential. When you reach a temporary plateau, remain patient and continue trying—proper training does not go unrewarded. You may want to try a few of the following techniques if you think you have reached a bit of a plateau:

- Try a couple weeks of easier training and stress reduction. Adjusting your training distance or intensity will often give you a new sense of vigour in training and racing. A new workout or route can often do the same.

- Review your dietary intake or see a registered dietitian for an analysis.

- Overhaul your entire training schedule.

- Re-evaluate your goals and set new ones.

# Overtraining

It is often during good weather, when we have a tendency to bump up our training distance because we enjoy being outside, that runners overtrain. The fatigue of overtraining is quite different from that felt from a week of hard training. Normal fatigue is relieved after a few days of rest or light training, but overtraining can last for months or longer.

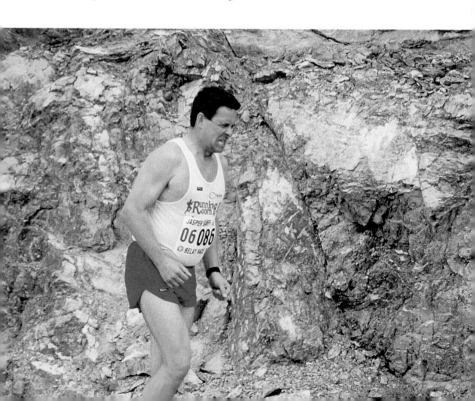

The symptoms of overtraining vary from person to person. The most common physical signs are:

- a rise in your resting heart rate
- decreased appetite
- a skin rash or sores in or around your mouth
- sudden weight loss
- a head cold or flu
- troubled sleep
- clumsiness
- swollen glands
- chronic muscle soreness
- decreased running performance.

Common psychological symptoms include:

- irritability
- depression
- anxiety.

If you have some of the signs of overtraining, back off the distance and intensity for a couple of days. A couple of easy runs combined with some extra sleep is normally a great way to energize your running, both mentally and physically.

To avoid the pit-falls of overtraining, return to the basic principles of training and plan your training program accordingly. Your body needs 36 to 48 hours to recover from a hard workout. You also need to have at least one full day of rest a week, and you should have extended periods of rest built into your long-term training program. There are two primary factors to consider when you plan your training program:

- to prevent injury and chronic fatigue, your program must allow adequate rest during heavy training;

- to detect overtraining, integrate performance and health evaluations into your program at times where normal fatigue won't be confused with overtraining.

A training log is an important tool for monitoring and avoiding overtraining because it keeps a record of the details of your training. Always remember the 10 percent rule: do not increase your weekly mileage by more than 10 percent a week, and do not increase the distance of your long run by more than 10 percent a week.

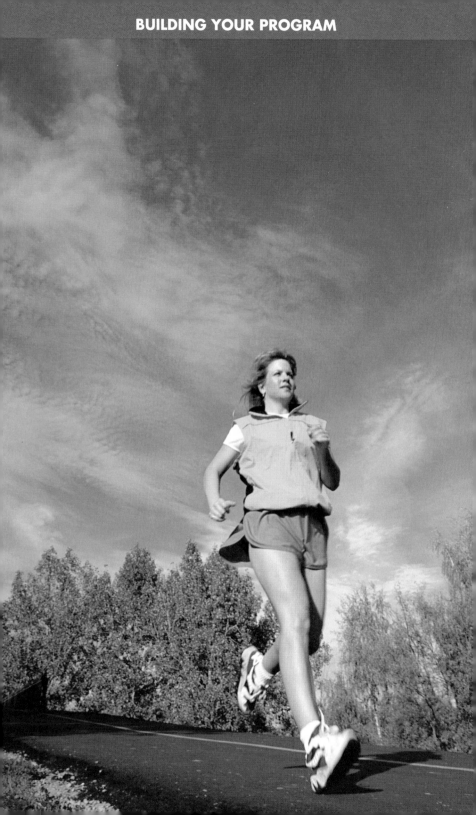

## Cross-Training

**Cross-training can often help you avoid overtraining—alternate exercises can give your body a break from running if you still want to get in some training.**

**Swimming**

**The buoyancy of the water workout is very gentle, and the swim stroke is good for stretching tight muscles.**

**Cycling**

**Spinning on a stationary or road bike is good therapy for tired legs. The non-weight-bearing action combined with easy spinning is a good way to alleviate any muscle soreness caused by hard running.**

**Walking**

**Yes, walking is a great alternative to running. Walking is a gentle way to loosen up sore, tired muscles when your legs are fatigued. Moderate to easy exercise will assist in the recovery of most muscle, tendon or joint stiffness.**

# Avoiding Injury

Runners quickly learn that the more they put into their sport, the more they get out of it. All runners, however, both advanced racers and beginners just setting out, have to be wary of injuring themselves. Relaxation and careful planning are the keys to enjoying your workouts and avoiding injury.

*Evaluate your fitness level honestly*

If you haven't been examined by a doctor lately, see one before you start running. Begin by running gently and walk when you feel tired. Remember, you should be able to carry on a conversation as you run. Be patient and only increase your effort after your body builds strength and adapts to the stress of running.

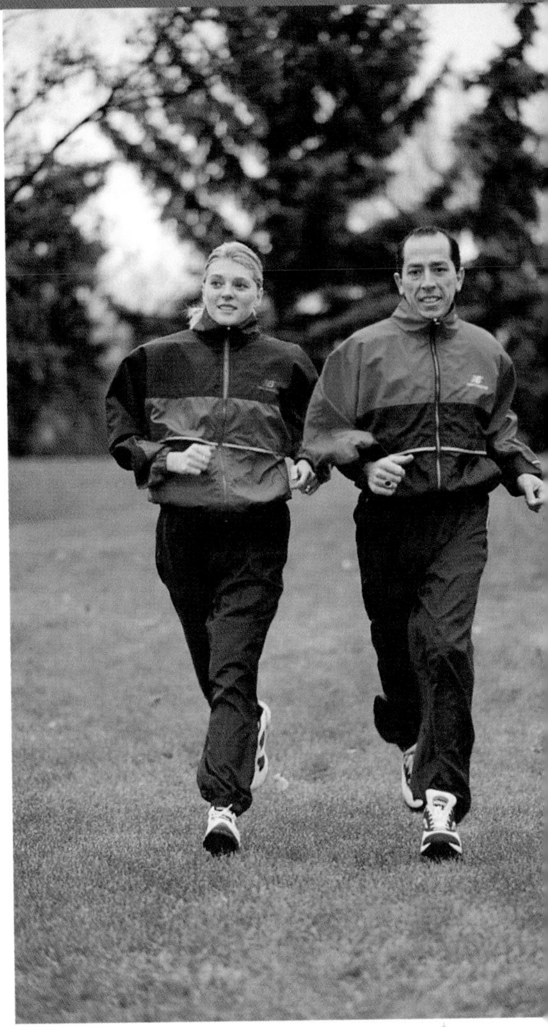

*Take your time*

Increase your training load by no more than 10 percent a week. For beginners, that means adding just a few miles a week to their weekly totals. It may not sound like much, but it will help keep you off the injured list so you can continue building. For instance, if you start with a base of around 20 miles (32 km) a week, in 10 to 12 weeks you can build up to 40 miles (64 km). That's enough to run a marathon, if that's one of your goals. You should also increase the distance of your long runs slowly—by no more than 2 miles (3 km) a week.

*Plan to plateau*

Don't increase your training load every single week. Once you've worked up to a comfortable level, stay there for three or four weeks before increasing again—gradually, of course. You could even choose to scale back periodically. For instance, after you build up to 14 miles (23 km) a week, you could run 10 miles (16 km) the following week before your next step up to 16 miles (26 km). Increasing your total distance every single week just won't work for long.

*Slow and easy does it*

Wait until you're completely comfortable with the amount of training you're doing before you start increasing your training pace, and even then, never speed up more than twice a week. As with distance, increasing your speed too much or too often can lead to injuries and fatigue. Be sure balance your speed workouts and long runs with slower, shorter days to give your body time to recover and build strength and speed. The same applies to racing, interval workouts and hill running.

*Focus on your running form*

If you concentrate on running with the best form, it can make your runs more fun because you won't be struggling against yourself. Besides, running with bad form can cause injuries: if you run too high on your toes or lean too far forwards, you can end up with shin splints or Achilles tendinitis; if you hold your arms too high or swing them back and forth too far, you can end up with stiff shoulders or an injured back.

For the most efficient running form, you should keep your body straight and lift your knees just high enough to let your legs swing forward naturally. Land gently on your heels and you'll have a productive stride that doesn't take too much energy. The focus of your running form should be the power coming from your hips and legs, with the rhythm and timing from a relaxed upper body.

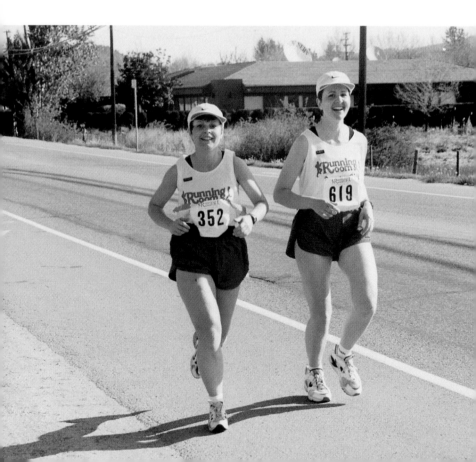

CH. 2

# TOP 10 LIST TO STAY FIT FOR RUNNING

1. Good running shoes.
2. A physical examination by your family doctor.
3. A sound training program.
4. Proper nutrition.
5. Adjust your training to the road surface.
6. Take it easy; run at a moderate pace.
7. Adjust your training to your conditioning.
8. Build into the intensity of your workouts and ease out of them.
9. Adjust the intensity and your clothing to the climate conditions.
10. Train at a pace that is consistent with your current level of fitness.

*Pay attention to nutrition*

Proper nutrition before, during and after each run will keep you more alert to your surroundings and your body's performance. Injuries often occur when a runner fatigues; good nutrition will delay this fatigue.

Everyone functions best on a diet that is high in complex carbohydrates, which means lots of fruits, vegetables, whole-grain products and low-fat dairy foods.

Foods to avoid include anything fried, pastries, cookies, ice cream and anything else high in fat. Replace sausage, bacon, untrimmed red meats and cold cuts with fish, lean red meats and poultry skinned and trimmed of fat. Wait 3 to 4 hours after a meal before running to avoid nausea and bloating. And don't forget those fluids, especially water—six to eight glasses a day are essential.

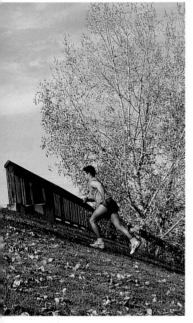

*Warm up before hill work*

Hills put a lot of stress on your cardiovascular system, so it's best to warm up for a few miles first to raise your heart rate more slowly. Once you start to climb the hill, shorten your stride, focus on lifting your knees and put more weight on the front of your feet. Pump your arms like a cross-country skier, keep your back straight, your hips in, your chest out and your head up, and lean forwards slightly. Don't go downhill too fast; it increases the chances of injury. Keep your arms low, tilt your body forward a little, stretch your stride a little and don't land too hard on your heels.

*Pay attention to those aches and pains*

If you want to avoid injuries and recover quickly, listen to your body. Interrupt your training program at the first sign of injury, even if you have to pass up a race—there will always be others. If your discomfort is mild and goes away—and stays away—during a run, it's probably OK to ignore it, but if a pain gets worse during a run or if it returns after each run, stop running. If you ignore your body's warning signals, you run the risk of developing much more serious injuries. Remember, pain is your body's way of warning you that something is wrong. Give your body a chance to rest—wait until your body is ready before you start running again. Once you've recovered, take it easy and slowly work back up to where you were. If you jump right back in at the same level, you're courting another injury.

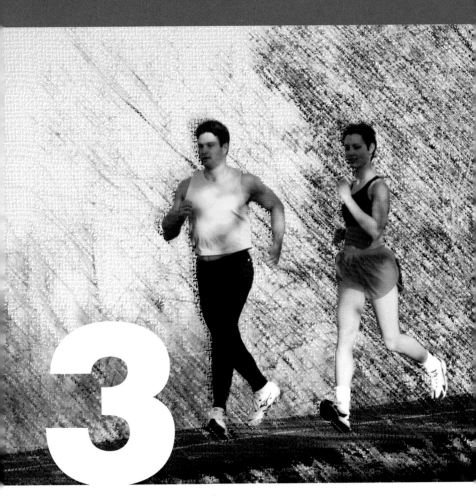

# 3

# Shoes and Clothing

## Selecting the Right Shoe

Shoes are a runner's most important piece of equipment—the average runner strikes the ground with a force of $3^{1}/_{2}$ to 5 times their weight, which has to be absorbed by the feet and legs—so you have to put some thought into which pair you choose. The right pair of shoes can enhance your performance and prevent injuries.

CH. 3

I have spent the past couple of decades around a running store, and I have seen many shoe models come and go—about every six months, the new, improved models replace the old. Some skeptics might tell you that it is all planned obsolescence, but I can tell you that there are folks running today thanks to the great improvements that have been made in shoe design and engineering. I have been to the research labs of some of the major shoe companies, and I have seen their rigorous testing programs—they are each trying to stay at the leading edge of design and technology. The entry-level shoes of today rival the top-of-the-line products of 5 or 10 years ago.

## Shoe Talk Terms

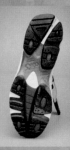

*Curved Last*

**Last: The form around which a shoe manufacturer builds a shoe. The average foot has a slight curve to it (about 7 degrees), and most shoes are built on a curved last to match this natural curvature. A shoe with a straight last has no curvature, which is suited to an overpronator with a low arch or flat feet.**

**Lasting: The method of construction used in joining the upper and the midsole of the shoe around the last. In a shoe with *board lasting* the upper is pulled over the last and the edges of the upper are attached to a piece of cardboard. The cardboard and the upper are then attached to the midsole. This shoe has good**

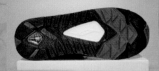

*Straight Last*

**stability but lacks flexibility. In *slip lasting*, the upper and midsole are sewn together around the last from the heel to the forefoot, which gives the shoe good flexibility but no stability. In *combination lasting*, the heel of the shoe is board lasted and the front is slip lasted, which gives the shoe good heel stability but allows for flexibility on toe-off.**

**Heel counter:** The stiff portion around the heel. It hugs the heel to give the shoe more stability and support. The further the heel counter runs along the medial side of the shoe, the more stable (and stiffer) the shoe.

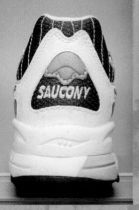

**Cushioning:** Each shoe manufacturer has its own system of cushioning—whether air, a gel, a liquid or a honeycomb of resilient materials—

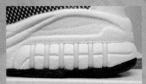

*Heel Counter*

to promote a soft, supportive ride in the shoe. The cushioning system is normally part of the midsole.

*Cushioning*

**Midsole:** Each shoe has a midsole that affects the stability of the shoe. The impact points on landing must be of a soft material to absorb the shock, and the control portion of the shoe must be of a greater density to adjust to the gait pattern of the runner. These aspects, together with the cushioning, give the runner a comfortable ride combined with motion control to enhance the runner's foot strike.

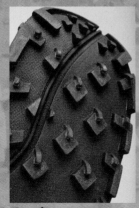

**Outsole:** The outsole, the bottom layer of the sole, can be designed for different running terrains. Some trail-running shoes, for example, have good grip for both going up and down slippery hills.

*Outsole*

# Three Types of Runners

The first step to choosing the right pair of shoes is to understand that runners can be grouped into three basic types: overpronators, normal pronators and supinators (under-pronators). Each type has specific shoe needs. As we run, our heel strikes the ground and our foot "pronates" by rolling inwards as the foot flattens out. The foot then "supinates" by rotating outwards after the weight is transferred to the ball of our foot. This great lever then becomes rigid and moves us forward.

**CH. 3**

## Overpronators

| Characteristics | Shoe needs |
|---|---|
| • Low arches. | • Straight last. |
| • Feet roll inwards too much: after landing on the outside of the heel, the weight shifts too far to the inside of the sole. | • Strong, rigid heel counter to keep the heel secure. |
| | • Medial and lateral support. |
| • Knees move inwards when the runner bends halfway at the knees. | • Firm midsole. |
| | • Wide landing base. |
| • Sole wears quickest on the heel, the centre and the inside of the forefoot. | • About 80 percent of technical shoes fall into this group. |

## Normal Pronators

| Characteristics | Shoe needs |
|---|---|
| • Normal, moderate arches. | • Semi-curved last. |
| • Feet hit softly on the heel and have a moderate degree of pronation. | • Moderate pronation control. |
| | • Moderate external heel counters. |
| • Knees stays neutral when the runner bends halfway at the knees. | • Durable midsole. |
| | • About 15 percent of technical shoes fall into this group. |

## Supinators

| Characteristics | Shoe needs |
|---|---|
| • High arches. | • Curved last. |
| • Lacks the normal inward rolling of the feet after the heel strike—the runner is in a supinated position during both landing and push-off. | • Moderate rear foot control. |
| | • Soft-cushioned midsole. |
| | • Light weight. |
| • Sometimes the heel wears quickest, but the wear pattern stays along the outside of the shoe. | • Low to moderate heel rise. |
| | • About 5 percent of technical shoes fall into this group. |
| • Knees move outwards when the runner bends halfway at the knees. | |

CH. 3

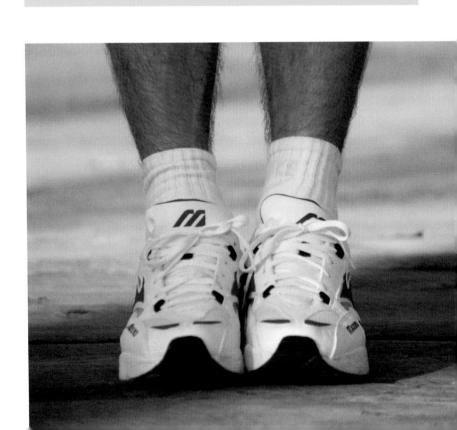

# Reading Your Old Shoes

Your old shoes reveal a lot about what type of runner you are, and if you walk into a good specialty store to buy a new pair of running shoes, a salesperson can often put you into the right pair in a matter of moments. Most magicians would never reveal the secrets of their trade, but I can take some of the mystery out of shoe selection with a few tips on how to read your old shoes.

View the upper of the shoe from the rear:

- The shoe's centreline should be perpendicular to the ground.

- The centreline shifts inwards, to the medial side of the shoe, if the runner has overpronated.

- The centreline shifts outwards, to the lateral side of the shoe, if the runner has supinated.

Check the condition of the midsole:

- The mid-sole compresses uniformly if the runner has normal pronation.

- The mid-sole compresses more on the inside of the shoe if the runner has overpronated.

- The mid-sole compresses more on the outside of the shoe if the runner has supinated.

Check the wear on the upper:

- The upper retains its shape if the runner has normal pronation.

- The upper sags inwards from the toe area if the runner overpronates during push-off.

# Shoe Buying Tips

When you go into a good specialty running store, you can be a little over-whelmed by the selection of running shoes. Today's shoes are very specific to individual runners' needs, so be sure to allow yourself enough time to choose the right pair. Here are some pointers to make your shoe-buying trip more productive:

**CH. 3**

- Take the time to consult with the salespeople at the store. They are generally runners who use the equipment daily in their own training and are in contact with other runners to get feedback on the latest models.

- If you're lucky enough to be in a store that can perform a video analysis of your gait and foot strike, take advantage of it—it's the best way to determine what you require in a shoe.

- Don't pick the shoe of your favourite running hero. Shoes are prescriptive, so find the shoe specific to your individual needs and requirements.

- Bring your old running shoes with you: an experienced shoe person can learn vital information from a worn pair of shoes.

- Take along your running socks so you are fitted in your new shoes with the same socks you will wear in training.

- If your wear an orthopedic device, take it along to be sure the new shoe has enough depth.

- Tell the salespeople how far you run in a week, what your running goals are, and about any injuries you have had, the type of terrain you run on and the kind of shoe that has worked for you in the past. This information can help them guide you to the right shoe.

- Good shoe folks will do a foot exam to determine your foot type and width. The more care taken by the shoe folks, the better the chances are you will be satisfied with the new shoe.

- Make sure the shoe fits the shape of your foot. Some shoes are narrow in the heel and wider in the forefoot; some shoes fit wide; some fit narrow. Work with your shoe selection to find the one that fits the most comfortably.

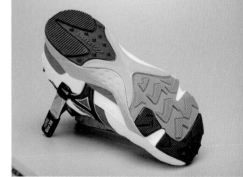

- You should lace up your shoes as you would boots or skates. The heel should be snug and there should be no movement in the heel when you walk or run—most shoes today have an extra eyelet hole at the top so you can get a snug fit in the heel. The breadth of the shoe in the forefoot should be snug without any pressure points.

- Once you have narrowed down the selection to a couple of different models, do the final test of walking and running in them. Good specialty stores will let you try out the shoes to see how they feel on a short run.

## Common Shoe Questions

### Can I run in my cross-trainers or do aerobics in my running shoes?

The answer is simply no. Shoes for running are designed for forward motion and for cushioning the impact specific to running. Other training shoes are designed for different specific uses. Aerobic shoes, for instance, are designed for lateral support and toe flexibility. Some cross-trainers are designed for running, but generally only at a moderate pace over a shorter distance. Spend the money on a good technical running shoe. It is one of the best investments you can make towards injury prevention.

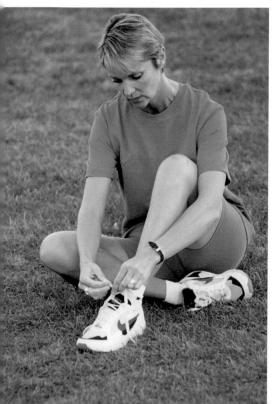

### How much should I spend on a shoe?

The price point for a good technical shoe starts at about $80 and goes up, depending on the amount of motion and cushioning control required for the individual runner. Pronation control shoes will generally cost a little more, because they require more technology in their construction.

### What is the average life of a running shoe?

Shoe manufacturers rate the average life of a shoe at about 500 to 700 miles (800 to 1100 km). Do not judge your shoes by the condition of the upper—the cushioning value is usually lost before the upper shows much wear. A good test is to try on a new pair of shoes to compare its cushioning to your pair's cushioning. You be the judge. Two key things to do are to mark the date you purchase new shoes and to keep track of the distance you run each day. Monitoring your distance and replacing your shoes frequently will keep you off the injury list.

**CH. 3**

### Do I need racing flats?

Racing flats are super light, which can increase a runner's leg turnover and bring down their 5-K or 10-K times. In coaching over the years, I have seen racing

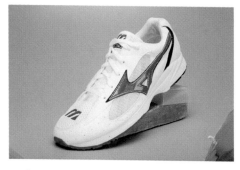

flats give runners an extra boost for a special race—that feeling of being extra light on your feet. Some models come with a small degree of support and stability for runners who overpronate, but I would not suggest a racing flat for a marathon. Unless you are planning on running a sub-2:40 marathon, the extra support and cushioning of a training shoe are far more important than the speed benefits of a racing shoe.

# Running Gear and Accessories

Besides shoes, there's an almost endless variety of clothing and accessories that can make your workouts more efficient and enjoyable.

## Clothing

**Socks:** Socks are important. After all, if your feet aren't comfortable, your run won't be, either. Socks range from the ultra thin and lightweight to those with a double-layer design that wicks away moisture and cushions your feet. Some socks have reflective lettering or markings on the ankle to help keep you visible after dark. Take along your shoes if you plan to try on socks, so you'll know exactly how they'll feel out on the road.

**Outer layer:** A good jacket can take you from fall through to spring if it's layered properly. Most importantly, you want a fabric that is windproof and breathable. Waterproof is also good. Vents along the back, zippered vents under the arms and adjustable sleeve cuffs allow you to control the amount of moving air you want on a particular day. Reflective strips are great for those winter runs

**CH. 3**

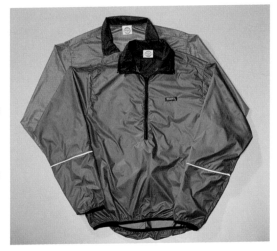

when the daylight disappears long before your run is over. Some jackets have a panel in the back that can drop down and cover your posterior, warding off the wind and rain, and a drawstring waist helps keep the wind out. Zippered pockets are also helpful to hold keys and change for an emergency phone call.

**Base, inner or single layer:** Forget cotton—it absorbs moisture and can cause chafing on longer runs. Look for synthetic fabrics designed to wick moisture away from the body. Polypropylene fabrics make a good base layer for cold-weather running. For hot weather, you might consider a fabric that offers UV protection. Women have a wide selection of tops to choose from, from tank tops that cover the entire midriff to tops with built-in support and cropped bra-style tops that also offer support.

**Pants and shorts:** Again, look for a fabric that wicks moisture away from the body, especially if you're wearing two layers in the cold. For a single or top layer, your pants can be either short for warmer weather, or long for the winter months. Some manufacturers put an extra layer along the whole front of the short for protection against wind, rain or snow when it's really cold. Some shorts for women have a tummy control panel.

**Middle or light top layer:** If it's really cold, a fleece top works well as a middle layer. Some fleeces, typically made with layered polypropylene, can act as a base and middle, or thermal, layer in one. If it's not too cold, a vest may be all you need as a top layer. Look for the same features you look for in a jacket.

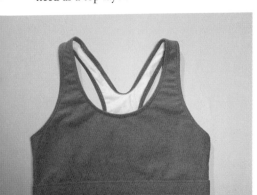

**Underwear for women:** A good supportive bra that offers motion control is essential for the female runner. Most major bra manufacturers make a sports bra; look for one with cushioned straps to disperse weight evenly and relieve pressure from the shoulders.

Some sports tops have the built-in support of a bra but can be worn as a single layer; there are even mesh sport tops for those really hot days.

**Underwear for men:** Men may want to wear a wind brief when it's really cold.

**Hats:** Fifty percent of the body's heat can be lost through the head during exercise in cold weather, so a hat that covers the ears is essential for a safe winter run. Fleece is a good hat material because it wicks moisture away from the head and is breathable. For really cold days, you can get hats that cover the whole head and ears, or even balaclavas, which cover the head and face, with cutouts for the eyes and mouth. If a hat is just too warm for you, try a band that fits around your head and over the ears. A hat is still a good idea for warm weather running, especially a baseball cap with a peak to offer protection from both the sun and rain. It should be made of breathable fabric that doesn't hold moisture.

**CH. 3**

**Mittens and Gloves:** Your hands do very little work to generate heat during running, so it is important to protect them from the cold. Fleece is a good material for mittens, especially if the fleece lines a windproof shell. Mittens are warmer than gloves, so for spring and fall you will want gloves that will keep your hands warm without making them sweat.

# Accessories

Now for the fun stuff. Good shoes and functional clothes are all you really need to run, but accessories can make your training time both more efficient and more fun.

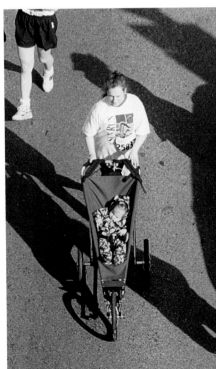

**Heart rate monitor:** Some of the better monitors are ECG accurate and offer wireless transmission from the chest unit to the wrist display. Look for monitors that are lightweight and waterproof. Basic monitors show your heartbeats per minute in a large, easy-to-read display; top-of-the-line monitors can record more than $2^1/_2$ days of information, including heart information every 5, 15 or 60 seconds, are programmable for multiple heart rate targets, and allow you to download the information to a personal computer.

**Sport stroller:** Having a young child is no excuse to miss a run—with an all-terrain, light and easy-to-handle sport stroller you

CH. 3

can take your child with you. Be sure to get a model with a canopy to protect your child from the sun and rain.

**Pedometer:** If you want to know how far you're running without having to measure your circuitous route on a map, a pedometer may be the answer. Electronic pedometers can be adjusted to your stride length to give you a reasonably accurate distance measure. Some models can also be used as a stopwatch.

**Music:** Lots of people like to run to music, and there are waist belts on the market that will securely hold your portable cassette or CD player for a jiggle-less run. You can also find special earphones that won't budge during your workout and have an easily accessible volume control on the connector cord. Just be sure not to listen to blaring music and run in traffic at the same time!

**Water belt:** Look for a lightweight belt that fits snugly around your waist so your water bottle won't jiggle uncomfortably. Belts can hold one or two water bottles, depending on the style, and some have zippered pouches for keys, change or food. If you like your water to stay cold, look for an insulated pouch.

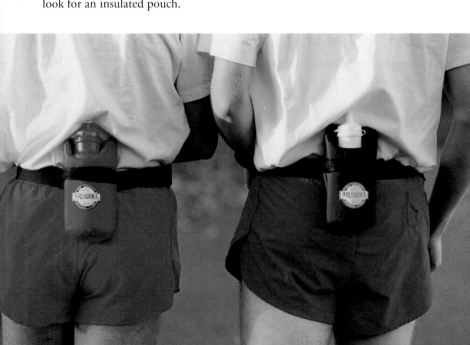

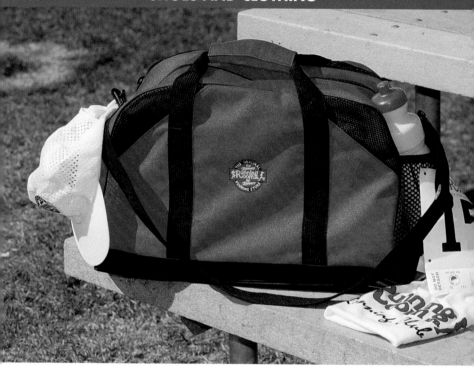

**Reflective clothing:** Working out after dark? Make sure you can be seen. Reflective clothing adds a measure of safety to your workout without adding a heavy layer.

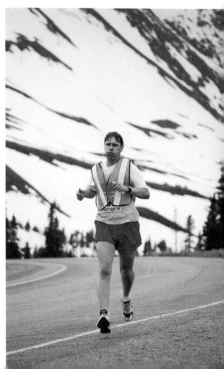

**Air-filter mask:** If you live in or travel to a city where air pollution is a concern, you may want to wear a mask to filter out pollutants and pollens—especially if you have asthma or allergies. Masks designed for athletes are the most comfortable to run in.

**Watches:** A runner's watch is essential to the runner in gauging the intensity and duration of their workouts. Timing your run/walk ratio and your recovery after the workouts can be managed with some of specific watches. Be sure to get one that is waterproof and readable in the dark.

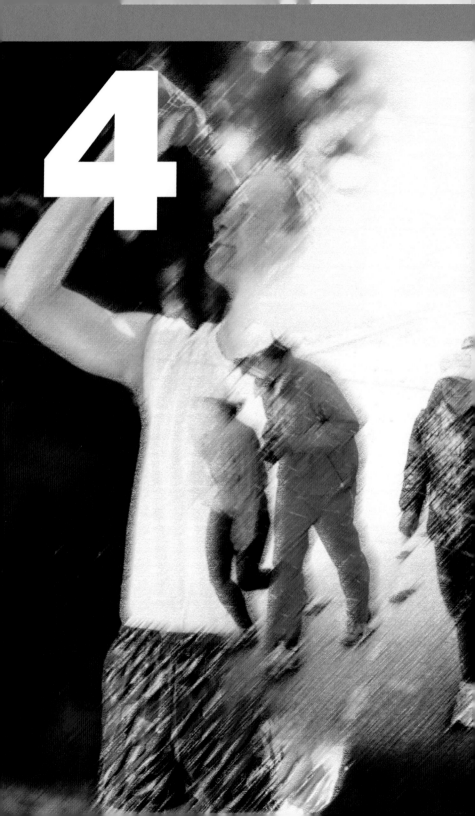

4

# Running Hot and Cold

## Cold-Weather Running

"Don't run out there or you'll freeze your lungs!"

Many of us heard those words as we were growing up, but, fortunately, there have been no documented cases of runners freezing their lungs. The biggest obstacle most runners have to overcome is their fear. For many people, the challenge is to convince or trick themselves into going outside on a blustery day. If your body is properly covered, the effort of running will soon warm you.

There is a special joy that comes from being the first person to make fresh footsteps through newly fallen snow. Build a snowman—it can become part of your cross-training regime to wake up your winter workout—and think of all of the character you are building as you head out on that long winter run. In the later stages of a future race, you can look back at the cold winter days you overcame with the wind blowing and the icy conditions. Heck, you can easily finish the last mile or so of that race.

## The Winter Workout

Icy road conditions, the risk of frostbite and longer periods of darkness create special concerns for winter runners, especially during severe winter conditions, but a little common sense and planning can make any winter workout safe and comfortable.

- Take the time to warm up adequately. You might stay indoors for the first part of your workout or do some on-the-spot running drills to elevate your heart rate.

- Start your run very slowly. Gradually increase the intensity in relation to the conditions: the colder the day, the less intense your workout should be.

- Check the direction of the wind. Run the first half of your workout into the wind so it will be at your back for the second half.

- Run a loop course, especially if you are running by yourself, so you can cut your workout short if the weather conditions worsen.

- Wear a reflective vest, reflective clothing, one of the small flashing runner's lights, a head lamp—whatever it takes—but keep yourself visible to others around you.

- Take enough water with you, the same as you would on a hot day. People often neglect proper hydration when it gets cold, but dehydration is still possible on a cold day, so take water on any run over 30 minutes.

- Take a sports nutrition bar on longer runs.

- Put petroleum jelly or a lip balm on the exposed skin of your lips and nose and around your eyes.

- Save your speed workout for a smooth, flat, well-lit and dry surface.

- Track runners use short sand runs to build lower leg endurance and strength; deep snow can give you the same benefits. With a little imagination, you can even visualize yourself running on a white-sand beach.

- Watch for the telltale signs of hypothermia so you can get yourself or your running buddy to a warm, dry place before you need medical attention.

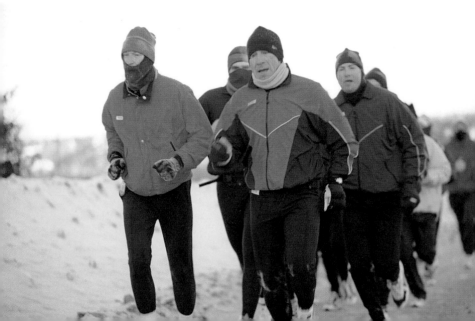

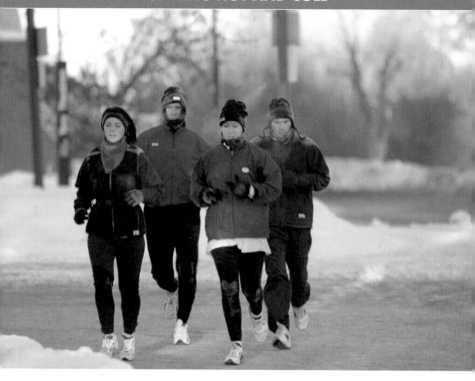

- Do not do any sudden accelerations or decelerations; it is very easy to pull a groin muscle or hamstring in cold weather.

- Turn corners slowly. If you keep your directional changes gradual, it will help you avoid a spill on the ice.

- Leave a map or note so someone will know where to look in case you run into trouble.

- Take along a few coins. An embarrassing phone call to a buddy for a ride beats a frostbitten nose. Cab fare can fit nicely under the insole of your running shoe.

- Run with a training buddy or with a group when possible.

- Run in well-travelled areas. A twisted ankle on a dark, snow-covered trail could leave you in serious trouble.

- An effective way to improve your footing and confidence is to twist some short metal screws into the soles of your running shoes. Come spring, they can be popped right out with very little trace of their winter holdings. (When I first suggested this one years ago, I got accused of spending far too much time outside.)

CH. 4

# Wind Chill

## Actual Air Temperature (° F)

| Calm | 40 | 30 | 20 | 10 | 0 | -10 | -20 | -30 | -40 |
|---|---|---|---|---|---|---|---|---|---|
| Wind Speed (m.p.h.) | Equivalent Chill Temperature | | | | | | | | |
| 5 | 35 | 25 | 15 | 5 | -5 | -15 | -25 | -35 | -45 |
| 10 | 30 | 15 | 5 | -10 | -20 | -35 | -45 | -60 | -70 |
| 15 | 25 | 10 | -5 | -20 | -30 | -45 | -60 | -70 | -85 |
| 20 | 20 | 5 | -10 | -25 | -35 | -50 | -65 | -80 | -95 |
| 25 | 15 | 0 | -15 | -30 | -45 | -60 | -75 | -90 | -105 |
| 30 | 10 | 0 | -20 | -30 | -50 | -65 | -80 | -95 | -110 |
| 35 | 10 | -5 | -20 | -35 | -50 | -65 | -80 | -100 | -115 |
| 40 | 10 | -5 | -20 | -35 | -55 | -70 | -85 | -100 | -115 |

## Actual Air Temperature (° C)

| Calm | 4 | -1 | -7 | -12 | -18 | -23 | -29 | -34 | -40 |
|---|---|---|---|---|---|---|---|---|---|
| Wind Speed (km/h) | Equivalent Chill Temperature | | | | | | | | |
| 8 | 2 | -4 | -9 | -15 | -21 | -26 | -32 | -37 | -43 |
| 16 | -1 | -9 | -15 | -23 | -29 | -37 | -43 | -51 | -57 |
| 24 | -4 | -12 | -21 | -29 | -34 | -43 | -51 | -57 | -65 |
| 32 | -7 | -15 | -23 | -32 | -37 | -46 | -54 | -62 | -71 |
| 40 | -9 | -18 | -26 | -34 | -43 | -51 | -59 | -68 | -76 |
| 48 | -12 | -18 | -29 | -34 | -46 | -54 | -62 | -71 | -79 |
| 56 | -12 | -21 | -29 | -37 | -46 | -54 | -62 | -73 | -82 |
| 64 | -12 | -21 | -29 | -37 | -48 | -57 | -65 | -73 | -82 |

| Apparent Temperature | Risk of frostbite |
|---|---|
| Above -20° F (-30° C): | Little danger |
| -20° to -70° F (-30° to -57° C): | Increasing danger—exposed flesh may freeze within 1 minute. |
| Below -70° F (-57° C): | Great danger—exposed flesh may freeze within 30 seconds. |

**Note:** Winds above 40 m.p.h. (64 km/h) have little additional effect.

# Hypothermia

**Hypothermia occurs when the core temperature of your body drops and your metabolic processes slow. There is fluid loss, your pulse rate drops and your equilibrium can be sent out of balance. It can be very dangerous. Symptoms are incoherent, slurred speech, clumsiness and poor coordination. Extra caution is necessary on cold, wet, windy days. At the first sign of hypothermia, get yourself or your training buddy to a warm, dry place. Seek medical advice and do not let the person fall asleep.**

## Cold-Weather Clothing

It is no secret that cotton is rotten for running: it holds onto your perspiration, and wet cotton is a poor insulator. The key to proper dressing in winter is to layer yourself with breathable fabrics that wick the moisture away from your skin, keeping you dry and warm. For a top layer, it's important to wear a jacket that is breathable but wind and water resistant. The best place to find the latest fabrics is at a specialty running store—some new synthetic fabrics have been created with runners and athletes in mind.

It is normal to feel slightly cold for the first 10 minutes of your run. Generally, you will warm up after that; in some cases you may even take off a layer on a longer run. Extra layers usually end up tied around your waist, so picking the right number of layers becomes a bit of a science. In most cases, it is better to be a little overdressed than under, because wind, rain or snow can change the conditions dramatically.

- A large proportion—up to 50 percent—of heat loss is through the head, so cover it up!

- Be sure that your hat covers your ears.

- Wear a balaclava to keep your head warm and covered in extreme conditions.

- Mittens, which allow for better circulation in your fingers, are warmer than gloves. Two layers of mittens work well on very cold days.

- Cover all areas of exposed skin with a breathable fabric to prevent frostbite.

- Under most conditions, three layers on the upper body and two layers on the legs will be more than adequate, providing the runner uses specific products designed for running.

- Start with a base layer of a synthetic fabric that will wick your perspiration away from your skin.

- Your shell layer should be pants or a jacket that again is a synthetic, breath able fabric, but wind and water resistant.

- Colder conditions call for an additional layer of fleece, or other synthetic, insulating fabric, between the base layer and the shell.

- Men may want to wear wind briefs. Their future generations will thank them and their post-race showers will be much more enjoyable.

- Wear socks made of polypropylene or another wicking, insulating fabric.

- Avoid wool. While it is warm, many people find it uncomfortable, and if it gets wet it becomes heavy and soggy.

## Heat Exhaustion and Heatstroke

**The early symptoms of both heat exhaustion and heat-stroke include hot and cold flashes, cold skin, dizziness, a decrease in the rate of perspiration, a headache or a build-up of heat in the head, confusion and disorientation. Heat-stroke can be fatal, so at the first signs of these symptoms, stop and get medical help immediately.**

## Hot-Weather Running

Running in warm weather is generally very pleasant and enjoyable, and the long summer days give us more quality hours in which to train. Pleasant as it is, however, you need to take extra precautions as the temperature and humidity rise. The clothing you wear and the fuel you feed yourself become important to your overall performance during a summer run. Good common sense in dealing with extreme conditions must be observed to avoid any opportunity for heat exhaustion or heatstroke.

- Take water on all your runs, regardless of the distance. Drink at least 2 cups (500 ml) of water for every 15 minutes of running.

- Water is the best fluid for runs lasting up to 3 hours. On longer runs, you may want to take an electrolyte drink, which will help replace the magnesium, Vitamin C and potassium that you have lost through sweating.

- Adjust the intensity and distance of your run relative to the heat. Slow down and enjoy the run: hot summer days are not the time to race, and you can always run long on another day.

- Run early in the morning. The coolest daylight hours are often just after sunrise.

CH. 4

- Remember: cotton is rotten for running. Cotton has a high sun protection factor, but it holds onto moisture, which reduces the cooling effect of evaporation. It also loses its softness when it's wet, which can case chafing. Save your cotton race T-shirt to wear while you brag about your latest run, not to actually wear running. There are some marvellous technical fabrics that will allow you to get the best in sun protection and stay as cool as possible.

- Check the UV index before you run. Sometimes, you may want the sun protection of a long-sleeved shirt, even in summer.

- Use sunscreen with a sun protection factor (SPF) of at least 30 on all exposed areas of skin.

- Chafing can be a problem for some runners. Use a petroleum jelly for the upper arms and thighs. Men should pay attention to their nipples; women should be watchful of the skin around the bra line, across the rib cage and under the shoulder straps.

- Do not drink alcohol before running in hot weather: it raises your metabolic rate and body temperature. A far better drink during the hot weather is skim milk. Save that glass of beer or wine for the celebration after the race or long run.

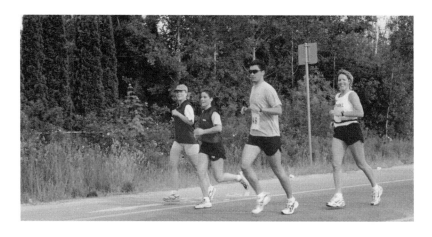

- If you enjoy a morning coffee, have an extra glass of water with it. Caffeine is a diuretic, so for those who drink it, moderation and additional water intake is very important.

- Wear a light-coloured, breathable fabric cap. Some models even have a flap that covers the back and sides of your neck.

- When you can, put some ice or a wet sponge under your cap to help keep your head cool.

- Splash yourself with water to help keep your body cool.

- Shorts made of technical fabrics, instead of cotton, will keep you both cooler and dryer and help prevent chafing.

CH. 4

# Heat Index

| | Actual Air Temperature (° F) | | | | | | | | | | |
|---|---|---|---|---|---|---|---|---|---|---|---|
| | 70 | 75 | 80 | 85 | 90 | 95 | 100 | 105 | 110 | 115 | 120 |
| **Relative Humidity** | Apparent Temperature | | | | | | | | | | |
| 0% | 64 | 69 | 73 | 78 | 83 | 87 | 91 | 95 | 99 | 103 | 107 |
| 10% | 65 | 70 | 75 | 80 | 85 | 90 | 95 | 100 | 105 | 111 | 116 |
| 20% | 66 | 72 | 77 | 82 | 87 | 93 | 99 | 105 | 112 | 120 | 130 |
| 30% | 67 | 73 | 78 | 84 | 90 | 96 | 104 | 113 | 123 | 135 | 148 |
| 40% | 68 | 74 | 79 | 86 | 93 | 101 | 110 | 123 | 137 | 151 | |
| 50% | 69 | 75 | 81 | 88 | 96 | 107 | 120 | 135 | 150 | | |
| 60% | 70 | 76 | 82 | 90 | 100 | 114 | 132 | 149 | | | |
| 70% | 70 | 77 | 85 | 93 | 106 | 124 | 144 | | | | |
| 80% | 71 | 78 | 86 | 97 | 113 | 136 | | | | | |
| 90% | 71 | 79 | 88 | 102 | 122 | | | | | | |
| 100% | 72 | 80 | 91 | 108 | | | | | | | |

## Actual Air Temperature (° C)

## Apparent Temperature

| Relative Humidity | 20 | 23 | 26 | 29 | 32 | 35 | 38 | 41 | 44 | 47 | 50 |
|---|---|---|---|---|---|---|---|---|---|---|---|
| 0% | 17 | 20 | 22 | 25 | 28 | 31 | 33 | 35 | 38 | 40 | 43 |
| 10% | 17 | 20 | 23 | 26 | 29 | 32 | 35 | 38 | 41 | 45 | 48 |
| 20% | 18 | 21 | 24 | 27 | 30 | 34 | 37 | 41 | 45 | 50 | 55 |
| 30% | 18 | 22 | 25 | 28 | 32 | 36 | 40 | 45 | 51 | 58 | 65 |
| 40% | 19 | 22 | 25 | 30 | 34 | 38 | 44 | 51 | 59 | 67 | |
| 50% | 19 | 23 | 27 | 31 | 35 | 42 | 49 | 58 | 67 | | |
| 60% | 20 | 24 | 27 | 32 | 38 | 46 | 56 | 66 | | | |
| 70% | 20 | 24 | 29 | 33 | 41 | 51 | 63 | | | | |
| 80% | 21 | 25 | 29 | 36 | 45 | 58 | | | | | |
| 90% | 21 | 25 | 30 | 38 | 50 | | | | | | |
| 100% | 21 | 26 | 32 | 42 | | | | | | | |

| Apparent temperature | Risk from prolonged exercise and/or exposure |
|---|---|
| 64° to 90° F (18° to 32° C) | Fatigue, dehydration possible. |
| 90° to 105° F (32° to 41° C) | Heat cramps or heat exhaustion possible. |
| 105° to 130° F (41° to 54° C) | Heat cramps or heat exhaustion likely; heatstroke possible. |
| above 130° F (above 54° C) | Heatstroke very possible. |

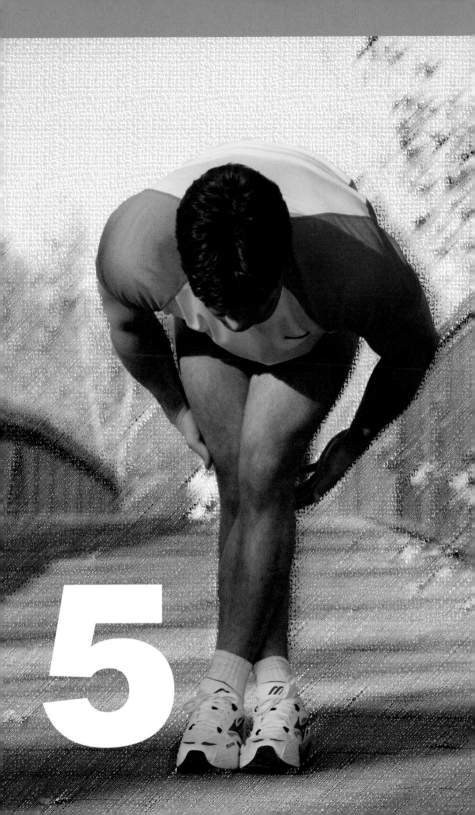

5

# Stretching

## Why Stretch

"Stretching? Well, maybe to get that last chocolate chip cookie on the far side of the table, but not for running."

CH. 5

A lot of runners will give you this kind of response when you ask about stretching. The debate on the benefits stretching has been going on for a while, between runners who follow a regular routine and runners who only do the occasional stretch as they blink away the previous night's sleep.

Studies by the sports medicine experts tell us that there is a correlation between injuries and stretching habits. They have found very little difference in injury rates between runners who stretch on a regular basis and runners who do not stretch at all, but runners who stretch occasionally have the highest incidence of injuries. In looking for a reason for their higher injury rate, they concluded that sporadic stretchers often stretch incorrectly and at the wrong time.

So, why stretch, you ask, when you can drop into a major road race and see some of the elite runners who can barely touch their toes without bending their knees? Well, remember that most of the elite runners did a good job in selecting their parents—pure speed has a lot to do with genetics—the rest of us need whatever other advantages we can find.

The thing I have found as I have aged from a runner to a coach is that maintaining flexibility is a real factor in maintaining some semblance of speed. Think of the two ways we run faster: a faster leg turnover and a longer stride. As we age, if we do not work at maintaining our flexibility, the stride length of your youth will soon leave us. Even if you are able to maintain your leg turnover, a shorter stride length means slower times.

The repetitive action of running causes the two major muscle groups, the hamstrings on the back of the thigh and the quadriceps on the front, to tighten up when put through the relatively limited range of the running motion. Stretching is integral to maintaining a full range of motion at the ankle, knee and hip.

Along with aerobic fitness and strength, flexibility should also be thought of as an important component of fitness and well-being. It has been generally believed that performing warm-up exercises that include stretching can help you

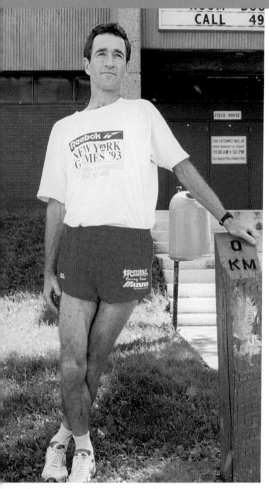

avoid injury during the subsequent activity. Although this may not be completely true, a well-planned warm-up, cool-down and stretching regimen are important aspects of every training session.

# When to Stretch

Stretching is always best done when the muscles are warm. If you prefer to stretch before you work out, then be sure to do a full 10-minute warm-up first. Alternately, you can make stretching part of an extended cool-down. If improved flexibility is your goal, then stretching while your muscles are cooling from a training session will give you the best results. Never sit down to stretch immediately after a workout; a proper cool-down is a prerequisite to the post-training stretch. No time after a workout? Try stretching during a shower or after a warm bath, when you are usually relaxed and your muscles are warm.

## Warm-up

The main purpose of the warm-up is to ready the body for the subsequent activity. It helps the heart, lungs and muscles prepare for exercise and eases the body through the transition from rest to exercise.

There are many forms of warm-up. Calisthenics, stretching and other forms of stationary exercise are popular. The best way to warm up is to do the planned exercise activity, only much more slowly for the first several minutes. For example, you can begin your run with a brisk walk, working up to a slow jog and then finally running. Tennis players often warm up playing at the service lines rather than using the full court.

How do you know if your warm-up has been long enough? Are you sweating yet? Perspiration is a sure sign that the warm-up can end and the training can begin.

## Cool-down

The purpose of the cool-down is to assist the body in the transition from exercise back to rest. It allows the heart to adjust to the decreased intensity gradually, and it can help prevent laboured breathing at the end of a higher-intensity session. Blood flow can slow more naturally during a cool-down, which will prevent the blood from pooling in the exercising muscles, thus avoiding the dizziness or nausea that can result from suddenly stopping an intense exercise.

**CH. 5**

As with the warm-up, the bulk of the activity done during the cool-down should be the same or similar to the training session, only slower or on a smaller scale—try to finish every run with a slow jog or a walk.

The optimum length of the cool-down is dependent on the intensity and duration of the prior exercise: longer, more intense training sessions require an extended cool-down period. A cool-down period of 5 to 10 minutes should suffice for most workouts.

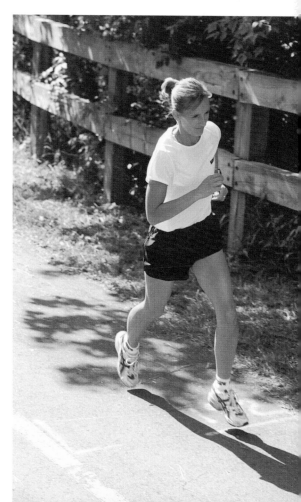

# Stretching Exercises

Here are the core stretching exercises you should be using as part of your program. Be sure to do both sides of the body, even if one is tighter than the other. And remember to think of stretching as one of life's pleasures.

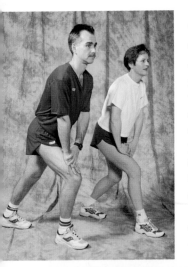

## Calf

There are two key muscles you are stretching in the calf area: the gastrocnemius is the large, heavy muscle below the back of the knee; the soleus is at the lower part of the calf above the heel. To do the stretch, stand about 3 feet (90 cm) from a wall or other support with your feet flat on the ground, your toes turned slightly inwards and your back straight. Lean into the wall and move one foot forwards, bending that leg at the knee. Gradually straighten the rear leg until you feel mild tension in the calf. Now drop the knee of the rear leg to stretch the area near the Achilles tendon. Switch legs and repeat.

## How to Stretch

Try to stretch the way you stretch when you wake up from a long sleep: a gentle "I feel good" stretch is your goal. Stretching should be done slowly and without bouncing. Be gentle on yourself: stretch to where you feel easy tension, but not pain. Any pain means you are hurting yourself. As you hold the stretch, the feeling of tension should diminish. If it doesn't, ease off slightly into a more comfortable position. After holding the gentle stretch, slowly move farther into the stretch until you feel mild tension again. This tension is where the muscles and tendons are making their adaptation. The feeling of tension should diminish slightly or stay the same. If the tension increases or becomes painful, you are overdoing it; ease off to a position that is more comfortable.

# Hamstrings

Sit flat on the ground with one leg out straight in front of you and the other leg bent at the knee and dropped to the side. Keeping your upper body straight, bend at the waist and move your head forwards over your straight leg. You do not need to touch your nose to your knee—or even be close. Some runners bend their back and then drop their head right down to the knee, but keeping the back straight helps isolate the specific muscles of the hamstring you want to stretch. Switch legs and repeat.

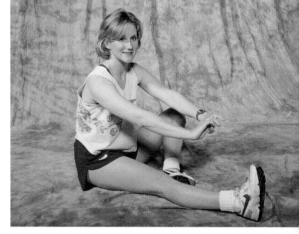

This stretch should be nice and gentle. No bouncing! Bouncing will engage the stretch reflex, which can actually tighten the muscle rather than extend it. For those runners looking for an option, this stretch can also be done with a towel hooked on your foot while you lay on your back.

# Quadriceps

Using one hand to balance yourself against a wall or other support, bend one leg at the knee and use your free hand to pull the foot up straight behind the leg; the foot shouldn't be pulled or pushed to the side. To protect your back during this stretch, be sure to pull in your abdominal muscles and keep your back straight. Switch legs and repeat.

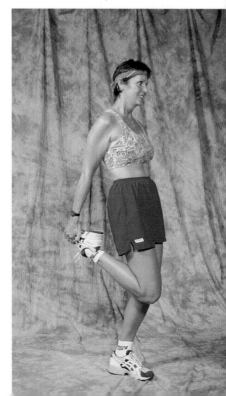

## Iliotibial Band

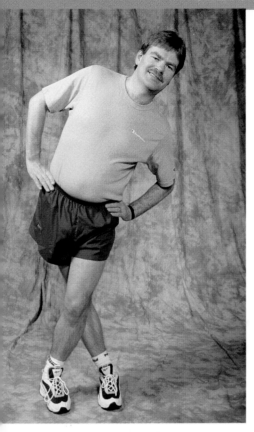

Stand parallel to a wall or other support. Keeping your upper body erect, bend your outer leg slightly at the knee, cross your inner leg behind it, and shift your weight so that your hip leans in towards the wall. You should feel the stretch over the hip area. Face in the opposite direction and repeat with the other leg.

## Buttock

Sit up straight on the ground with one leg out straight in front of you and of the other leg bent up at the knee. Cross the foot of the bent leg to the outside of

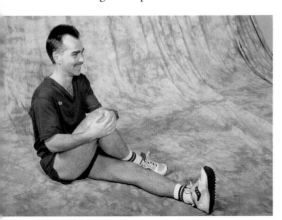

the straight leg. Slowly pull the bent knee in towards the opposite shoulder. You will feel the stretch in the buttock of the bent leg. Switch legs and repeat.

## Hip Flexor

Kneel on one knee and place the other foot forward, flat on the ground so that the leg is bent at a 90-degree angle. Keeping your back straight, your abdominal muscles pulled inwards and your rear knee firmly planted on the ground, move your hips forwards. You should feel the stretch in the hip of the rear leg. Switch legs and repeat.

CH. 5

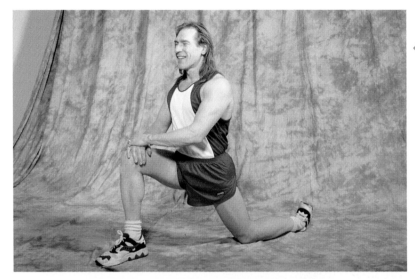

## KEYS TO BETTER STRETCHING

- Stay relaxed.
- Only hold the stretch tension that feels comfortable.
- Keep your breathing regular—don't hold your breath.
- Don't worry about how far you can stretch.

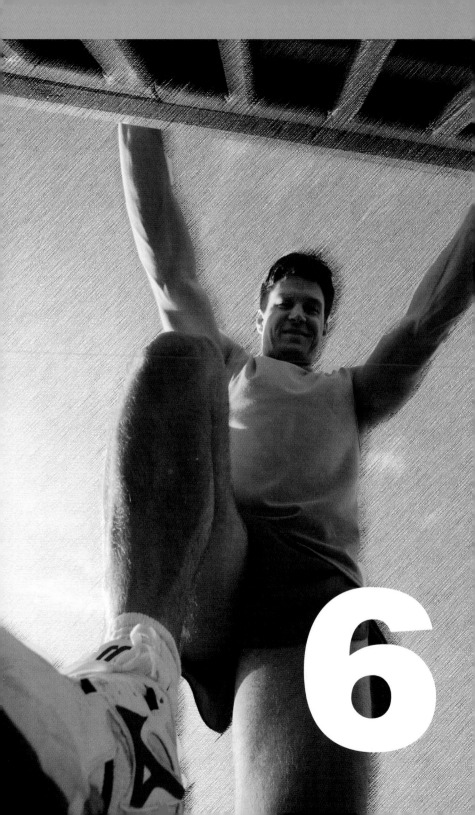

6

# Introductory Training Programs

So you've decided to take up a healthier lifestyle and you've chosen running as your means of getting there. Making that decision is a big step, but the hardest part of getting started is making the initial commitment to yourself. The real secret to staying committed is to make your program gentle enough for your current physical condition and yet challenging enough that you will see some progress.

Chapter 10 (Nutrition) goes into the details about how to fuel that athletic body you're going to have, but for now just focus on these key points:

- Drink 8 to 10 glasses of water each day.

- Cut down on the amount of fats and oils in your diet.

- Increase the amount of complex carbohydrates in your diet.

## Smart Running

**Guidelines for street-wise runners and walkers:**

- **Carry identification or write your name, phone number and blood type on the inside of your shoe or in a running shoe key holder that attaches to the outside of your shoe.**

- **Don't wear jewellery.**

- **Carry change for a phone call.**

- **Run with a partner whenever possible.**

*continued...*

75

*...continued*

- **Write down or leave word of your running route. Tell your friends and family of your favourite routes.**

- **Run in familiar areas. Know the locations of telephones and open businesses and stores. Alter your route.**

- **Always stay alert. The more aware you are, the less vulnerable you are.**

- **Avoid unpopulated areas, deserted streets and over grown trails. Especially avoid unlit areas at night. Run well clear of parked cars and bushes.**

- **Don't wear headphones. Use your ears to be aware of your surroundings. If you just can't run without music, use earphones that still let you hear what's going on around you.**

- **Wear reflective material if you must run before dawn or after sunset.**

- **Use discretion in acknowledging strangers. Look directly at others and be observant, but keep your distance and keep moving. Ignore verbal harassment.**

- **Run against traffic so you can observe approaching automobiles.**

- **Use your intuition about suspicious persons or areas. React to your intuition and avoid any person or area that feels unsafe to you.**

- **Carry a whistle or a noisemaker.**

- **Call the police immediately if something happens to you or someone else, or if you notice anyone out of the ordinary during your run.**

# Walk Before You Run

Just how do you get started if you've basically been a sedentary adult who has done nothing in the way of physical activity? The following walking program is a gentle way to get started and is normally acceptable to most people. The mistake that most people make in getting started is going too far, too fast and with too much intensity. Fitness is a lifetime goal, so be easy on yourself to start with and keep the intensity gentle.

This program is measured out in minutes to help you manage a low-intensity workout. Sports medicine experts tell us that as little as 20 minutes of activity, three times a week, is a good way to get started and is also a good way to maintain cardiovascular fitness.

CH. 6

This program gives you one day of rest after each workout. Rest is part of the program, and it is important that you treat rest as part of your training. Patience is also part of the program. A healthy lifestyle is a long-term commitment, and you have lots of time to attain that goal. This program will help you progressively and cautiously improve your current fitness level.

## Preconditioning Phase

During this phase, concentrate on time, not intensity, in your walks.

| | Mon | Tues | Wed | Thurs | Fri | Sat | Sun |
|---|---|---|---|---|---|---|---|
| Week 1 | rest | walk 25 min. | rest | walk 20 min. | rest | walk 25 min. | rest |
| Week 2 | rest | walk 25 min. | rest | walk 20 min. | rest | walk 30 min. | rest |
| Week 3 | rest | walk 25 min. | rest | walk 20 min. | rest | walk 35 min. | rest |
| Week 4 | rest | walk 25 min. | rest | walk 20 min. | rest | walk 40 min. | rest |
| Week 5 | rest | walk 25 min. | rest | walk 20 min. | rest | walk 45 min. | rest |
| Week 6 | rest | walk 30 min. | rest | walk 25 min. | rest | walk 45 min. | rest |
| Week 7 | rest | walk 35 min. | rest | walk 30 min. | rest | walk 45 min. | rest |
| Week 8 | rest | walk 40 min. | rest | walk 35 min. | rest | walk 45 min. | rest |
| Week 9 | rest | walk 45 min. | rest | walk 40 min. | rest | walk 45 min. | rest |
| Week 10 | rest | walk 45 min. | rest | walk 45 min. | rest | walk 45 min. | rest |

Congratulations! You are now into some real fat-burning exercise. In just 10 weeks, you have progressed from being a sedentary person to being an athlete who gets in three, 45-minute fat-burning sessions a week. Now you will really start to see an improvement in your fitness.

This is a good time to talk about the scale. Many people become slaves to weighing themselves when they start a fitness program. My suggestion is to only weigh yourself at the start of the program, so you know your starting point. Rather than using weight as a measurement of your progress, it is better to use the fit of your clothing. Take a pair of pants and a shirt that fit before you start your program, and try them on each week to see how they loosen up as your fitness improves. Watching your clothes slowly become baggy can be very motivating, and it keeps you away from the scale, which sometimes only shows how much water you've been drinking.

CH. 6

## Endurance Phase

Now that you are comfortable walking for 45 minutes, three times a week, it's time to combine some faster walking with slow, recovery walking. This is not power walking or race walking, but a series of timed intervals: intensive phases where you simply walk faster, followed by recovery phases where you walk slower.

|  | Mon | Tues | Wed |
|---|---|---|---|
| **Week 11** | rest | 10 min. warm-up; 3 min. fast; 3 min. slow; 3 min. fast; 3 min. slow; 3 min. fast; 3 min. slow; 10 min. cool-down | rest |
| **Week 12** | rest | 10 min. warm-up; 3 min. fast; 3 min. slow; 4 min. fast; 4 min. slow; 4 min. fast; 4 min. slow; 10 min. cool-down | rest |
| **Week 13** | rest | walk for 60 min. | rest |
| **Week 14** | rest | walk for 70 min. | rest |

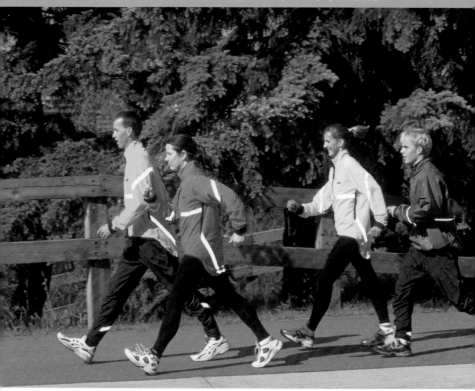

| | Thurs | Fri | Sat | Sun |
|---|---|---|---|---|
| | walk for 45 min | rest | walk for 50 min. | rest |
| | walk for 50 min. | rest | walk for 60 min. | rest |
| | walk for 60 min. | rest | walk for 75 min. | rest |
| | walk for 80 min. | rest | walk for $1^1/_2$ hr. | rest |

Wow! Now you're up to 1¹/₂ hours of calorie-burning exercise. As an athlete, you've learned how much fun and enjoyment you can get from an intelligent training program. Now you're probably ready to start training as a runner.

# Beginner's Conditioning Program

Once you can walk briskly for 30 minutes, you can start interspersing some easy running into your walking. By slowly exchanging running for walking over several weeks, you will gradually progress to non-stop running.

## Training Rules

- **If you can't keep up or lose time from illness or injury, don't panic. Stay at the level you can handle or go back to a level until you are ready to move on.**

- **Remember: it took a lot of years to get out of shape, so take your time getting back into shape.**

- **Your goal is to run 20 minutes non-stop—smiling and talking all the way. It doesn't matter if you take 6 weeks or 4 months to reach that goal.**

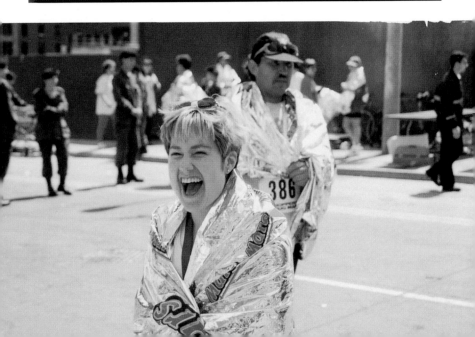

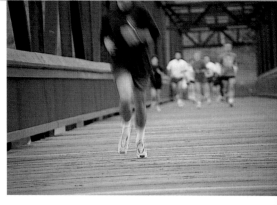

The following schedule should be run at least three times a week. All running should be done at a conversational pace, meaning that you can easily talk while running, and all walking should be done briskly. Of course, a proper warm-up and cool-down are required. This program starts conservatively, so if you fall behind a little, you can easily get back on track. Once you reach the halfway mark, however, you may find it difficult to keep up unless you run faithfully at least three times a week, and preferably five.

CH. 6

| Week | Run-walk training session | Total run time |
|:---:|:---:|:---:|
| 1 | run 1 min., walk 2 min., x 6 sets; run 1 min. | 7 min. |
| 2 | run 1 min., walk 1 min., x 10 sets | 10 min. |
| 3 | run 2 min., walk 1 min., x 6 sets; run 2 min. | 14 min. |
| 4 | run 3 min., walk 1 min., x 5 sets | 15 min. |
| 5 | run 4 min., walk 1 min., x 4 sets | 16 min. |
| 6 | run 5 min., walk 1 min., x 3 sets; run 2 min. | 17 min. |
| 7 | run 6 min., walk 1 min., x 3 sets | 18 min. |
| 8 | run 8 min., walk 1 min., x 2 sets; run 2 min. | 18 min. |
| 9 | run 10 min., walk 1 min., x 2 sets | 20 min. |
| 10 | run 20 min. non-stop | 20 min. |

# Intermediate Conditioning Program

If you can currently run for 20 minutes, with a walking break or two, a couple of times a week, you are ready for the intermediate program. This program starts off with a few weeks of walk/run training to assist you in the transition to regular run training.

CH. 6

| Week | Training session | Sessions per week |
|------|------------------|-------------------|
| 1 | run 5 min., walk 1 min., x 4 sets | 3 |
| 2 | run 7 min., walk 1 min., x 3 sets | 3 |
| 3 | run 10 min., walk 1 min., x 2 sets | 3 |
| 4 | run 20 min. non-stop | 3 |
| 5 | run 20 min. non-stop | 3 |
| 6 | run 22 min. non-stop | 3 |
| 7 | run 24 min. non-stop | 3 |
| 8 | run 26 min. non-stop | 3 |
| 9 | run 28 min. non-stop | 3 |
|   | run 20 min. non-stop | 1 |
| 10 | run 30 min. non-stop | 3 |
|   | run 20 min. non-stop | 1 |

Once you are running for 30 minutes, three times a week, don't increase the length of those training sessions, but concentrate on gradually bringing your running time up to 30 minutes on your fourth weekly session. You are progressing well, and you don't want to risk injury, fatigue or boredom.

# Advanced Conditioning Program

If you can currently run for 20 minutes or longer, non-stop, on a consistent basis, you are ready for the advanced program. This program focuses on safely increasing your total running time as well as adding extra training sessions each week.

| Week | Running session | Sessions per week |
|------|-----------------|-------------------|
| 1 | 20 min. non-stop | 3 |
| 2 | 22 min. non-stop | 3 |
| 3 | 24 min. non-stop | 3 |
| 4 | 26 min. non-stop | 3 |
| 5 | 28 min. non-stop | 3 |
| 6 | 30 min. non-stop | 3 |
|   | 20 min. non-stop | 1 |
| 7 | 30 min. non-stop | 3 |
|   | 22 min. non-stop | 1 |
| 8 | 33 min. non-stop | 3 |
|   | 22 min. non-stop | 1 |
| 9 | 33 min. non-stop | 3 |
|   | 24 min. non-stop | 1 |
| 10 | 30 min. non-stop | 2 |
|   | 25 min. non-stop | 2 |
|   | 20 min. non-stop | 1 |

CH. 6

After you have reached week 10, when you are running five times a week, hold your longest runs at 30 minutes and concentrate on gradually bringing your other runs up to 30 minutes as well. You don't want to risk injury, fatigue, or boredom.

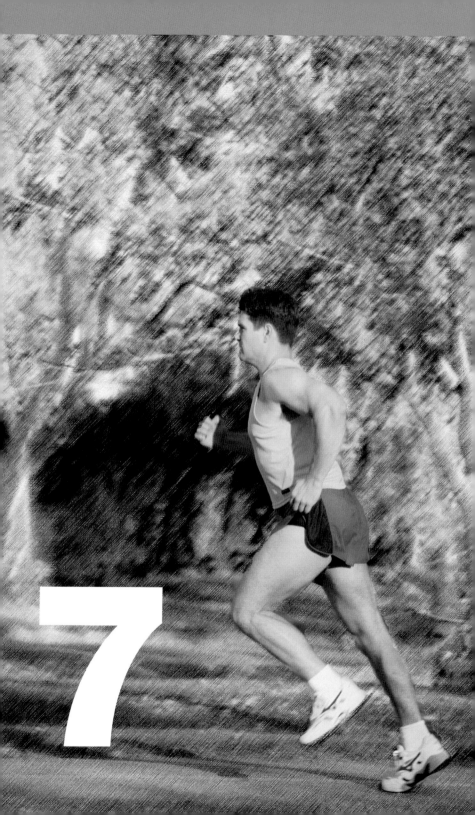

7

# Running Form

*How can I improve my form?* is one of the most frequent questions coaches hear. If you don't have a coach, one of the best ways to assess your running form is to review a video of yourself running—we are often our own best critics when we see ourselves on tape. If you can't get a video, ask a running buddy for an objective assessment.

Before getting into a discussion on form or giving advice to a trainee, I usually suggest that they come with me to the finish area of a local road race, so they can watch the lead runners come in. It is always very apparent that in the lead pack, as in the whole pack, there are some runners with great-looking form and then there are some with butt-ugly form. What I ask the trainee to look at is not the display of form as much as the degree of relaxation. The lead runners are certainly fast—after all they are in the lead at the finish—but if you study their concentration, you can see that they maintain a more relaxed form even under race conditions.

Another thing to do is to go down to a local track area and listen to the advice of the running coach. The number one thing you will hear the coach say during a workout is, *Relax*. The coach will be making all kinds of points to the runners, but the basic thing the coach wants the runners to do, no matter how hard they are pushing, is to relax.

So relax, and let's take a look at how to improve your running form.

## Posture

A relaxed, upright posture is the simplest body position. Getting your head, shoulders and hips lined up over your feet just makes it easier to move the whole body forwards. It's also easier to breathe in that position. The lungs are being used to their maximum efficiency when they are not constricted in any way. Stand tall, with your shoulders relaxed, and keep your mouth slightly open and your face relaxed. Smiling will help relax your face—it also confuses your running competitors. Weight training that involves any of the muscles that affect posture, including your shoulders, abdominals and lower back, will also help.

## Breathing

When it comes to breathing, swimmers are the best athletes to study; if they make a mistake, it means getting a mouthful of water. Swimmers learn to be rhythmic with their breathing, keeping it in time with the rate of exertion: the harder and faster the swim, the more the air the swimmer needs. It sounds simple enough.

Many runners have the problem of breathing backwards: they suck in their abdomens and breathe in with their chests. Switch to belly breathing; it gets you breathing with your lower diaphragm so your lungs can inflate fully. If you master this breathing technique, you can stay more relaxed and in control of your running form.

## Hips and Chest

CH. 7

First, imagine that you have a button in the middle of your chest. It's attached to a string that leads up a hill in front of you and is pulling you along the road. Next, shift your hips forwards to keep the alignment right in your posture. Strong abdominal muscles will help maintain this form—here is a reason for those sit-ups.

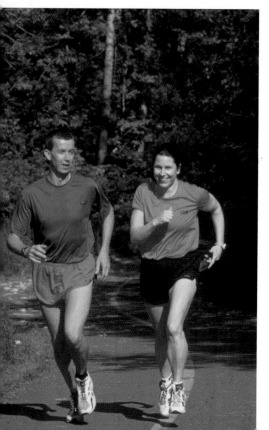

## Leg Turnover and Stride Length

There are two ways to increase your speed in running: increase the distance covered in each step (your stride length) or increase the number of steps you take in a minute (your leg turnover). In attempting to increase your stride length, it is very easy to over-stride, which can actually slow you down with the extra pounding and braking effect. Apart from hill running, where you should shorten your stride on the uphills and lengthen your stride on the downhills, let your legs choose their own stride. Do whatever comes naturally and lets you stay relaxed. The proper stride length

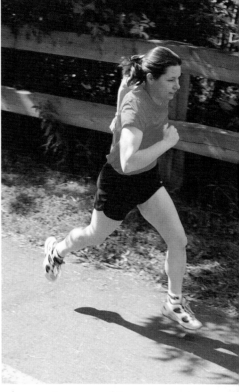

will keep you smooth and relaxed in your run, with your feet low to the ground, allowing you to increase your leg turnover if you want to speed up. Try to lead with your knees; it will keep your alignment correct and help you concentrate on the correct push-off.

## Foot Strike and Push-off

Running experts now recognize that we really can't mess too much with a runner's foot strike: some runners land on the heel and then transfer weight to the toe for push-off; some land on the forefoot and push off directly; some land with a ball/heel action. Like your fingerprints or maximum heart rate, these are gifts from your parents. What we can do is make the most of the gifts we have been given. When it comes to foot strike, the most important thing to try to find is the sweet spot where the reflex action and the power push are happening together. Practise some accelerations and you will soon find the best combination of your stride length and the timing of the push from the ankle as it shifts forwards.

## Ears and Eyes

What do ears and eyes have to do with running? They can dramatically improve your running form and efficiency. Use your ears to listen to the sound of your feet hitting the ground. Practise some accelerations or listen to the sound during a normal run. Now try to run as quietly as possible, staying as light as you can on impact. You will find that this exercise will improve your leg turnover and running form. Another trick is to watch the road ahead of you and notice how the horizon bounces as you run. Try to run with as little bounce as possible, which will get you into a more efficient, shuffling run. Sprinters run with more knee lift and height—power running is faster over short distances—but most runners will benefit from taking as much bounce out of their forms as possible.

# Look Ma, No Arms!

"When I'm running, I'm never sure just what to do with my arms."

If you hear yourself in that statement, you're not alone. Take a look at a group of runners, and you will notice that everyone has a different arm carriage and arm swing: some runners carry their arms up high like a shadow boxer; others carry their arms low and have very little arm swing; some arms are loose and relaxed; others are tight. Proper arm carriage is more efficient, so it will allow you to run faster with less effort; the key to efficient arm movement is the same as for many other aspects of running form: stay relaxed.

Let's start with your hands. To relax them, try touching your thumb and middle finger lightly. You will notice that this relaxes the palm of your hand. Now think

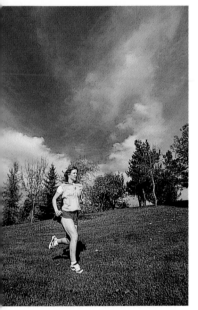

about keeping your wrists loose and relaxed. Keep the palm of your hand down as you run, and don't clench your fists. One trick to teach you to relax your hands is to run holding saltine crackers in your hands. They should still be whole at the end of the run.

If you can keep your hands relaxed and as loose as possible, you will find that your forearms and upper arms also stay relaxed. We have all seen people running along with their arms dangling, trying to loosen up their shoulders. The reason that most of them end up with tightness in their shoulders is that they have been running with clenched fists. The tightness that starts in your hands and forearms works its way up the arms into the shoulders. Staying relaxed can easily prevent this discomfort.

The next thing to consider is arm swing. Think about where your heart is located and the fact that it has to pump blood to all parts of your body—all the major muscle groups are looking for additional blood during running. As far as your hardworking heart is concerned, the most efficient place to carry your arms is in the area of your heart, so keep your arms bent at about 90 degrees. If you carry your arms too high, the blood has to be pumped uphill; if you carry your arms too low, the heart has to pump the blood a further distance.

Remember that running is a forward-motion sport; try to keep all your movements in the same direction as your running. I like to think of my arms as a metronome that keeps the timing and rhythm of the run smooth.

Your body type and running gait also govern your arm motion. You will see elite runners like Bill Rodgers who sometimes have one arm with a flick of outward motion. When I asked Bill why he runs this way, he told me it is because one of his legs is slightly shorter than the other. Our bodies adapt very quickly to irregularities, and Bill's arm flex is its way of compensating to keep his running form efficient.

Track coaches work hard with their athletes to keep their arms under control and efficient; if you think your arm carriage needs some work, here are a couple of arm drills that might help. (Some runners find these drills awkward; they prefer to just focus on keeping their arms and hand movements smooth and rhythmic when they run, and not to cross the centre line.)

## Apple Pocket Drill

Think of reaching for an apple, placing the palm of your hand over it, pulling it back and putting it in your pocket. The palming motion of your hand over the imaginary apple gets you to relax your hand. Bringing your hand back towards your pocket keeps your movement in your line of motion. Work at keeping your hands really loose, and practise clipping your hip with your thumb on the way.

The tightness that develops between the shoulders in many runners is often the result of running with clenched hands and tight forearms—the tension travels up the arms and settles in between the shoulders. This drill will help keep you relaxed and loose in the upper body.

## Hands and Arm Drill

This drill is one you have likely seen track athletes working on, running and slicing the air with their hands. Think of a line drawn though the centre of your head and body down between your legs; you want to keep your arms from crossing over this line. If your arms cross over too far in front of your chest, the lateral motion causes your lower back to tighten up. Try standing on the spot and work your arms in a running motion. If you exaggerate the cross-over motion you will feel the stress that it puts on your lower back. Think of running as a forward-motion sport—keep your movements efficient by concentrating on this in all your motions. Relaxed arm swing keeps your upper body relaxed while improving your form and ease of breathing.

CH. 7

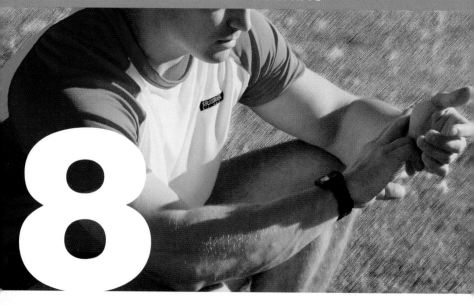

# Heart Rate Training

Different training workouts require you to exercise at different intensities (see chapter 9 [Types of Running]). As your training intensity increases, so does your heart rate, and monitoring your heart rate is probably the most widely known method of determining your training intensity. The development of wireless heart rate monitors has given many athletes, from beginners to experts, an easy, effective way to gauge their training intensity.

You can't always predict how your heart is going to respond to exercise. Fatigue, illness and overtraining can have profound effects on heart rate, so always listen to your body. Don't be a slave to your heart rate monitor; you should look at it about every 10 minutes—not every minute—especially during a race.

## Understanding Training Intensities

Depending on the intensity of the exercise, our bodies will supply energy to working muscles by aerobic metabolism, anaerobic metabolism or a combination of the two. "Aerobic" and "anaerobic" are two terms that are thrown around quite loosely on the track and in the gym these days, but a lot of people don't really understand them.

"Aerobic" means "in the presence of oxygen"; when the intensity of exercise is such that there is enough oxygen to supply energy by aerobic metabolism, it is called "aerobic exercise." Aerobic metabolism can supply energy for hours on end, because it is quite efficient and only very small amounts of lactic acid form during aerobic exercise, so this byproduct can normally be removed from the muscles before any ill effects, such as stiffness or soreness, are felt. The drawback of aerobic metabolism is that it is relatively slow; most people can supply energy by predominantly aerobic metabolism for intensities corresponding to up to 60 percent of their maximum heart rate. This limit, however, is highly trainable.

"Anaerobic" means "in the absence of oxygen"; when the intensity of exercise is too high for the body to get enough oxygen, and aerobic metabolism is too slow to supply energy at such a fast rate, the body must shift gears and produce energy by anaerobic metabolism. Such high-intensity exercise is called "anaerobic exercise." Anaerobic metabolism can supply energy at a very fast rate and requires less oxygen, but the chemical reactions involved produce large quantities of lactic acid as a byproduct. Lactic acid is produced faster than the blood system can remove it from the muscles, and if enough lactic acid accumulates in the muscles, it can cause a burning sensation in the legs and a queasy feeling in the stomach. If anaerobic metabolism continues, so much lactic acid will accumulate that it will interfere with the energy-making process and the exercise will have to slow or come to a complete halt (whether you want it to or not). For this reason, anaerobic metabolism can continue for only a couple of minutes. Yes, only two!

CH. 8

"Anaerobic threshold" is an important concept to understand, because much of your training will revolve around it. Your anaerobic threshold is the point at which the intensity of an exercise becomes too great for aerobic metabolism to supply energy fast enough for the demands of the exercise. A gradual shift to anaerobic metabolism occurs to support the increased energy demands, and lactic acid starts to accumulate in your muscles.

A key point to understand about aerobic and anaerobic exercise is that there is no activity that can be defined as entirely one or the other—most activities that we participate in require both types of metabolism. For example, although the marathon is predominantly and aerobic activity—it requires a steady output of energy over a long period of time—there are still aspects of the event that require anaerobic metabolism.

# Determining Maximum Heart Rate

Heart rate training requires you to know your maximum heart rate, which very few people do. Very few athletes have the opportunity or the motivation to take part in a physiological test to exhaustion—the proper way to determine your maximum heart rate—so we must have an alternate method that will estimate our maximum heart rate with some accuracy. Good luck! Very few researchers and exercise physiologists can agree on the most appropriate method for estimating maximum heart rate. Remember that whatever method you use to estimate your maximum heart rate, there is always a degree of error. Use your results only as a guideline; the important thing is to listen to your body when you train.

There is a very simple and commonly used predictive formula for your maximum heart rate: if you are a man, subtract your age from 220; if you are a woman, subtract your age from 226. For example, a 40-year-old man would have a maximum heart rate of about 180, and a 40-year-old woman would have a maximum heart rate of about 186.

## Heart Rate Formula

**Estimating your maximum heart rate**

**Men: subtract your age from 220**

**Women: subtract your age from 226**

A more practical test for estimating maximum heart rate is the maximal hill run. To perform this test you need the following:

- A heart rate monitor.

- A hill of approximately a 10-percent grade and 600 to 800 metres long. (It should take you 3 to 5 minutes to climb the hill at your maximum pace—no longer!)

- The conviction that you can push yourself to maximum exertion. It is difficult, but you only have to do it once. Plan on doing a high-quality, high-performance workout that is quickly over.

After an appropriate warm-up of at least 10 minutes (that includes stretching), make your way to the bottom of the hill. Run as hard as you can to the top of the hill without stopping. (Remember, it's not an all-out sprint; it will take some pacing.) At the top, check your heart rate monitor. You should be pretty close to your maximum heart rate. Don't stop running at the top—you have just run really hard and taxed your anaerobic metabolism, so there will be a lot of lactic acid in your blood and muscles. An active recovery phase will help remove the lactic acid from your system. Be sure to do a proper cool-down, including stretches.

This type of test definitely takes some practice, which means you may have to do it more than once to get the best results. Be sure you are completely recovered before doing another maximal hill run. You may even want to try it on another day.

# Using your Monitor while Training

## Base Training

Your base training should be at 50 to 70 percent of your maximum intensity. For example, if your maximum heart rate on the hill test is 180 beats a minute, then during your long slow runs your heart rate should be no higher than 126 beats per minute. Typically, runners find it difficult to keep their heart rate below the limit they have set. Doing the long runs at an agonizingly slow pace is the toughest component to teach most athletes, but they must learn. The whole purpose of long slow runs is to build endurance and stamina. Strict training in this area will prevent you from losing steam in the last few miles of your long run.

CH. 8

## Threshold Training

The purpose of this type of training is to work on proper form, strength and endurance. Set a target heart rate of 75 to 85 percent of your maximum heart rate for your threshold training sessions. A good guideline, in most cases, is to run at your 10-K race pace. You are not going to do this type of run every day—hill training is an example of a threshold workout—and any more than a couple of times a week will over-fatigue your legs and compromise your long run.

## Speed Training

Because of their intensity, speed training runs are best done as interval training. This is speed—high quality stuff requiring 85 to 100 percent effort in relation to your maximum heart rate. Speed training is a high-quality session, not high-quantity, so your intervals should be no longer than 7 to 12 minutes. As with hill workouts, start off with only two or three and build slowly. Your heart rate should recover to approximately 120 beats a minute after 1 or 2 minutes of rest before starting the next interval. Vary the distances of the intervals and the total distance of the workout from week to week. With this type of training, a warm-up and cool-down are critical: for each, do 2 miles (3 km) of easy running and a stretch.

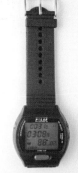

# The Heart Rate House

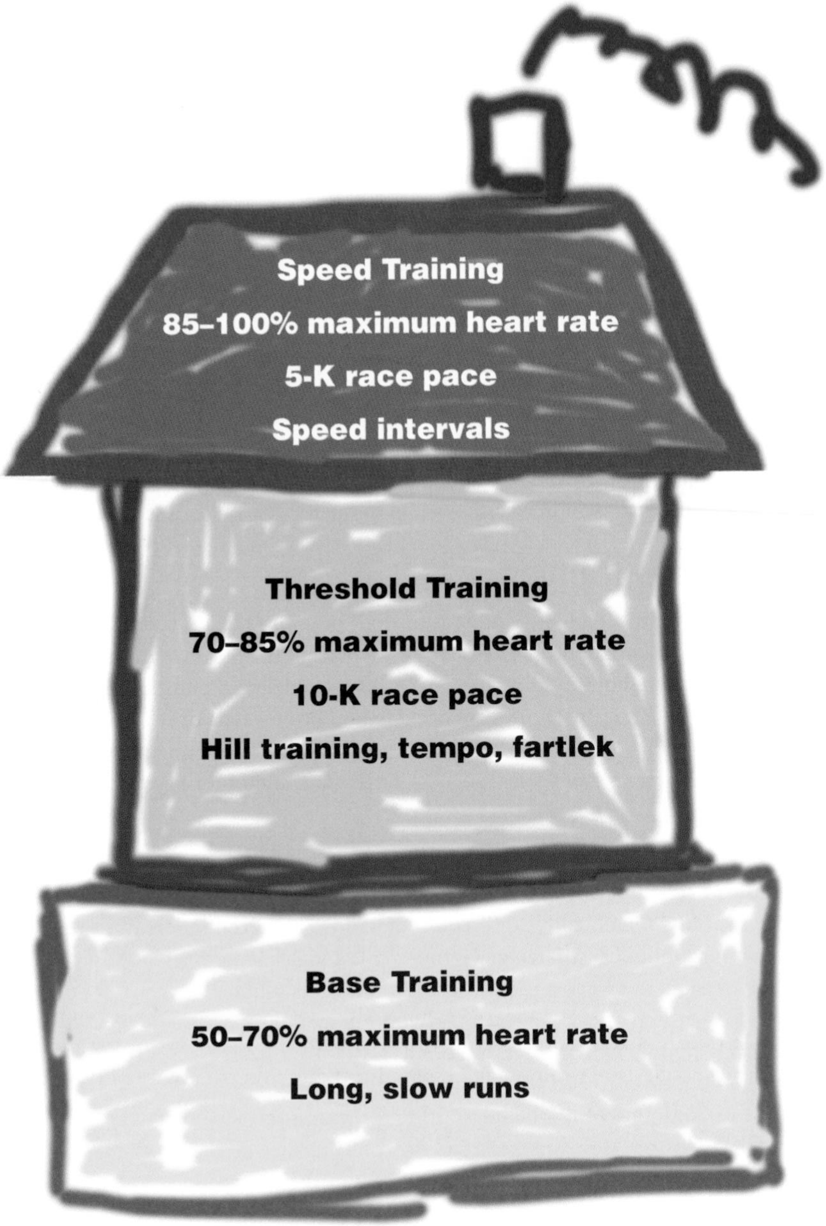

**Speed Training**

**85–100% maximum heart rate**

**5-K race pace**

**Speed intervals**

**Threshold Training**

**70–85% maximum heart rate**

**10-K race pace**

**Hill training, tempo, fartlek**

**Base Training**

**50–70% maximum heart rate**

**Long, slow runs**

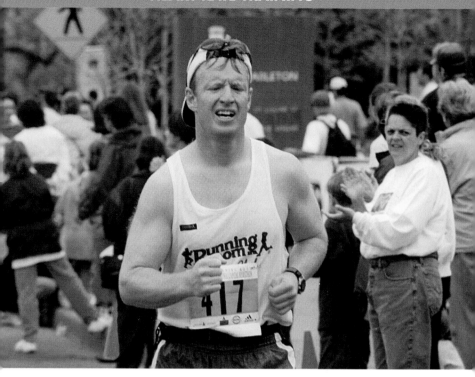

# Using your Monitor while Racing

If you start a race at an even pace, it should take at least 3 minutes to get to your steady-state heart rate. With that in mind, you can use your heart rate monitor to keep from starting out too fast.

For shorter events, such as a 5-K or a 10-K, have a plan before you get started about your target heart rate for the different stages of the event.

For events lasting longer than 1 hour, such as a marathon, half-marathon or 10-miler, you must be careful when using a heart rate monitor because of a phenomenon known as cardiovascular drift, which is common in long events. Cardiovascular drift is characterized by an increase in heart rate without an increase in intensity. The heart rate can 'drift' higher during these long events because of dehydration, over-heating or fatigue. Marathoners have observed as much as a 15-beats-per-minute increase in heart rate over the course of the race, even though their pace remained the same. Runners who maintain their heart rate religiously during these long events will only find themselves going slower if they don't allow for a gradual rise in their heart rate.

# Monitoring Overtraining and Rest

As a recreational runner, you may not think that you are a candidate for overtraining syndrome, but overtraining does not discern between recreational and elite athletes. In fact, elite athletes often have coaches and trainers monitoring every aspect of their training, so it is highly unlikely that they will overtrain. The runners who are most susceptible to overtraining are the highly motivated runners who try to perform during every training run and competition. (See "Overtraining," p. 35, for more details.)

Changes in your resting and exercise heart rates can be early signs that you're beginning to overtrain. Monitor your resting heart rate in the morning before you get out of bed. Be sure to do it on those days when you can sleep until you wake, rather than when the alarm clock bolts you upright. A consistent and significant rise in your resting heart rate is a sign that your body is fatigued or that an illness is impending. Exercise heart rates in the overtrained state are not as predictable. Many overtrained athletes experience decreases in their exercise heart rate (as you would expect with training), which may be due, in part, to their inability to maintain training intensity due to fatigue. In other athletes, however, overtraining can cause an increase in their training heart rate. In any case, your best defence against overtraining is to listen to your body and plan appropriate amounts of rest in your training program. Use your heart rate monitor as an overtraining prevention tool.

CH. 8

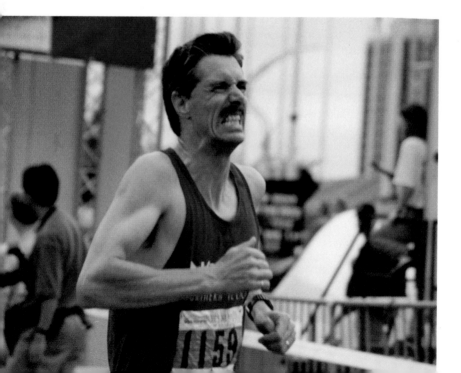

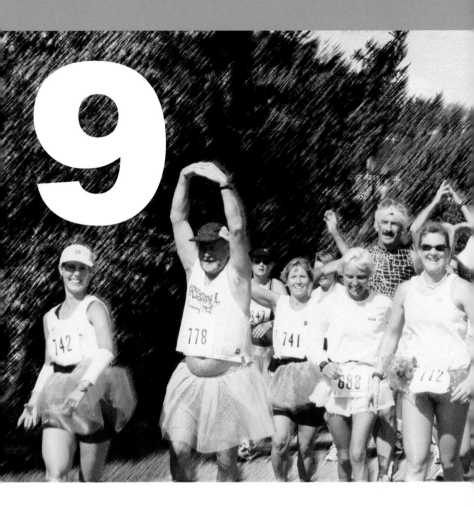

# Types of Running

Basic running is as simple as putting one foot in front of the other—quickly—but there are various kinds of running that can be used for different purposes: speed work, for instance, such as interval training and fartleks, helps a runner run faster; hill work builds strength; long runs build endurance. This chapter looks at the various types of running and how you can incorporate them into your training program.

| Run Type | Description |
| --- | --- |
| Continuous run (easy) | Steady run below targeted race pace. |
| Continuous run (race pace) | Steady run at or above targeted race pace. |
| Tempo run | Long repetitions at targeted race pace or faster with recovery intervals in between.<br>e.g., 3 reps. of 2000 m at 10-K race pace / 5–7 min. recovery rest, walk or jog. |
| Intervals (speed) | Fast runs over short distances with recovery jog intervals in between.<br>e.g., 8 reps. of 400 m fast run / 400 m recovery jog. |
| Intervals (strength) | Faster runs over shorter distances with shorter recovery jog intervals in between.<br>e.g., 12 reps. of 300 m fast run / 100 m recovery jog. |
| Fartlek | Change-of-pace runs of various distances of the runner's choosing (continuous running in bursts).<br>e.g., 45–50 min. fartlek: warm-up; 4 reps. of 50 m fast / 50 m jog; 5 min. steady; 1200 m fast; 10 min. steady; 3 reps of 400 m fast / 400 m jog; 4 min. steady; 1 mi. easy. |
| Long run | Longest runs of your training program; steady, continuous run lasting at least 70 min. |
| Base mileage | Shorter endurance runs done on your easier days. |
| Hill repeats | Repeated runs up and down a hill. Run hard going up; easy coming down. |
| Surges | Short intervals at race pace spread out over a continuous run.<br>e.g., 4–8-mi. (6.5–13-km) run with 1–6-minute bursts at targeted 5-K or 10-K pace. |

CH. 9

## Purpose

To develop stamina and build strength.

To develop stamina and pace judgment. Improves your confidence.

To develop strength, speed and pace judgment. Simulates race conditions in a condensed version.

To develop speed, raise anaerobic threshold and improve leg speed and coordination.

To develop strength and speed, raise anaerobic threshold and improve cardiovascular system.

CH. 9

To build determination, strength and speed. Teaches the athlete to shift gears between training speed and race speed.

To increase capillary network in your body and raise anaerobic threshold. Mentally prepares you for long races.

To raise your basic metabolic rate and increase anaerobic threshold "Massage" runs teach you that a gentle run improves your recovery from a hard workout.

To develop strength. Helps teach pacing to the runner who has a tendency to go out too fast.

To develop strength and speed. Add spark to your speed sessions but are so short they are fun.

# Hill Training

Hill sessions are intense workouts that build your lower leg strength and improve your running form without the pounding of speed. The intensity of a hill workout can vary from 70 to 85 percent of your maximum heart rate during the uphill phase; you should recover to about 120 beats per minute between hills. Choose an intensity based on your current fitness level: not so fast that you have to stop part-way up; not so slow that you recover well before you reach the bottom again. Make sure you are not tired from your previous day's run; you should be fully prepared to work hard.

## Hill training builds character

**As you do the hill repeats, say to yourself, either mentally or verbally, "character." Repeat it over and over. On race day when you discover a hill on the course, think back to the hill sessions and repeat the word "character." Take comfort from the fact no race course will have 12 hills in it.**

Here's how to do it:

- Pick your hill: it should have an incline of 8 to 10 percent, and it should have a length of about 400 metres if you are training for a marathon or half-marathon, or about 200 metres if you are training for a shorter event.

- Warm up with about a 2-mile (3-km) run.

- Now, to get up that hill, you'll probably have to use a little bit of visualization. Look at the top of the hill and visualize the hill as flat. Don't run with your head down—your eyes should be focused on the top of the hill, just as they would be focused in front of you on a flat stretch.

- The first thing to concentrate on is form. Keep your chest up and out and your breathing relaxed. Think of the power coming from your legs, strong and efficient. Your arms should always be in rhythm with your legs. Your arms won't actually propel you up the hill, but they can help you maintain proper form and leg speed. When your legs start to slow near the top, pump your arms a little faster and your legs will follow.

- The key is to maintain the same effort as you go up the hill. Shorten your stride as the hill gets steeper—your speed will slow slightly—and increase it again as you reach the crest of the hill. Keep up the same effort and run past the top—don't stop!—before turning around.

- As you run downhill, don't lean back or put on the brakes; it will only slow you down and risk injury. Instead, consider gravity your training buddy: open your stride a little, lean slightly forward and away you go. Gravity will speed you up with no additional effort on your part.

- Start with 4 hill repeats and increase by 1 repeat each week, to a maximum of 12 repeats. Allow at least two days of recovery after a hill session before you attempt another tough workout.

- If you run your hill sessions with a group, remember that this is your workout and yours alone. Do the warm-up and the cool-down with the group, but conquer the hill at your own speed.

- Think of driving a car with cruise control: as the slope of the hill increases, so does the throttle. Like the cruise-controlled car, you want to maintain a smooth powerful flow up the hill, which helps you learn the importance of pacing and effort adjustment.

CH. 9

## Hill Training Rules

- Warm up for 20 minutes and cool down for 10 minutes.

- Start with 4 repeats.

- Don't go beyond a maximum of 12 repeats.

- Keep an erect posture.

- Imagine that the hill is flat.

- Follow your hill workouts with 2 days of easy running.

Hill work builds strength in the quadriceps and the calf muscles and prepares you for the next phase of quality speed. Hills also build your confidence level, increase your self-esteem and prepare you mentally to be a better athlete. Come race day, the experience of the hill sessions pays big dividends as you pass runners not only going uphill but at the crest and going downhill, too.

# Running Drills
## (Teaching a Duck to Dance)

For years, Olympic coaches have been using running drills that focus on the muscles and tendons specifically used in running. The exercises develop the full range of motion of the leg, from push-off to the carry-through; they work the calf and lower leg muscles, the hamstrings and the quadriceps, along with improving running form and coordination.

Over time, most runners develop a much-improved cardiovascular system, but many lack overall coordination, flexibility and strength. The rewards of "going for a run" sometimes work to the detriment of your overall fitness as you over-develop the specific muscles used in the running motion. Running drills will improve your general athletic performance, and you will become a more powerful and efficient runner, which simply means that you will be able to run farther and faster with less effort.

CH. 9

The other thing running drills can bring to your training program is some fun. If you go to a playground, you can watch the sheer joy of children running and playing. Running drills should be approached in the same manner; they are going to add value to your overall conditioning and they can give you some variety in your running to keep it fun.

RUNNING DRILL RULES

- Be gentle in your whole approach to the drills.
- Think of the coordination involved, as well as the strength.
- Keep it fun. This is not work, it is play. Enjoy yourself.

The following drills are a high-quality workout for your running program, so approach them slow and easy. Find a smooth, flat surface to do these drills, either a rubberized track, a football field or even a smooth dirt trail, and do them with a noncompetitive group that can have some fun with the workout.

Some of the drills require good coordination, so if you find yourself struggling with one of them, skip it for now. Redoing a drill to try to get it right will only over-stress your body. Over time your coordination will improve. Even if you feel like they are trying to teach a duck to dance, you can take heart; improvement will come with practice.

Start with two repetitions of each drill and add one a week as your confidence and timing improves. After a few weeks, you can incorporate the drills into your warm-up for hills or speed intervals.

## Warm-up

• Start with an easy run to gradually warm up your system.

• Do some gradual accelerations over 25 to 50 metres to loosen up your muscles.

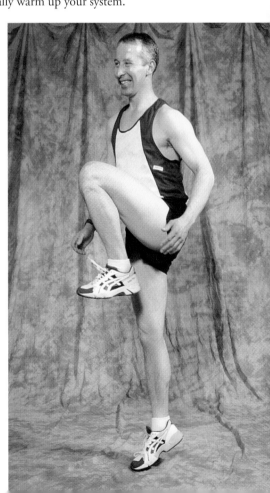

## High-knee Drill

This drill will work your feet, ankles, Achilles tendons, calf muscles, abdominals and the driving muscles in your butt. Take it easy, this is high-quality stuff. In addition to all of the muscle groups, you should also be working on your rhythm and coordination.

• Start with high-knee walking, lifting your knees as high as you can.

• Keep your posture erect.

• Drive your knees forwards to waist height.

• Rise up on your toes.

- Lean slightly forwards, but keep your posture erect.

- Think of the lift coming from your abdominal muscles.

- Start with a distance of 25 metres; gradually work your way up to about 100 metres.

- Think of a slow-motion action.

- Progress to high-knee running.

- Foot strike is quick and light—you are on hot coals!

- Think high knees and fast reflex action—you are prancing.

## Kick Some Butt

Ah ha, this sounds like just the kind of drill you've be looking for to vent some of that non-running stress. Well, I have some good news and some bad news: the good news is that you get to kick some butt; the bad news is that it's your own butt you'll be kicking.

**CH. 9**

The purpose of this drill is to primarily work on your body position while improving your coordination and flexibility. We have all seen runners who seem to sit back as fatigue sets in during the later stages of a long run. This drill will help you attain a slight forward lean, which improves your form and ultimately your running times by getting that old buddy gravity to do some of the work for you.

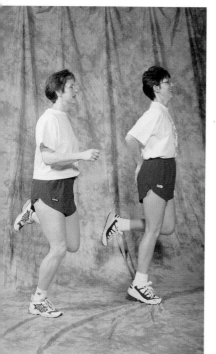

- Look slightly in front of where you are running.

- Keep your arms and hands loose at your sides.

- Get up on the front of your foot.

- Run with your feet kicking back.

- Try to kick high enough to kick your own butt, so to speak.

- Do repeats of 50 to 75 metres.

- Your arms will help to balance you, although it will feel awkward at first.

## Yahoo Jump

Most of us can recall this one from our youth. If we had done 20 of these a week, we would have developed all of the running muscle groups well, particularly the hip flexors.

• Stand with your feet together, flat on the ground.

• Jump forwards, keeping your feet together.

• Kick both legs forwards.

• Land with your feet together.

• Swing your arms to assist in the jump.

• Do a total of about 75 to 100 metres.

• Holler a loud *Yahoo!* (optional).

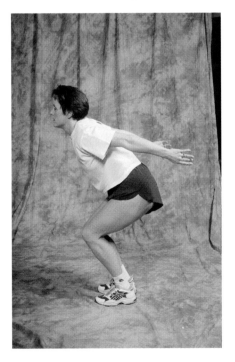 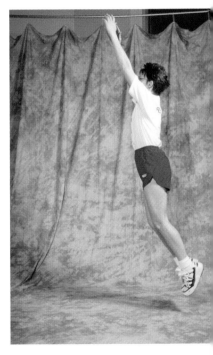

## Old Goose-step Drill

This is no Mother Goose drill; it looks easy, but once you try it you will discover that it's a great workout for your feet, ankles, quadriceps and hamstrings.

- Run up on your toes.

- Kick your legs forwards, keeping them straight.

- Keep your knees locked.

- Your arms should be bent at a 90-degree angle.

- Keep your steps short and fast.

- Chase the old goose for only about 50 to 100 metres; remember, you're looking for quality, not quantity.

## Pedal-to-the-Metal Bursts

This drill is a fun power acceleration in which you start slowly and then continuously accelerate for 100 metres. Try to maintain the form and coordination that you have been practising in the other drills. Relax, keep your breathing regular and concentrate on a steady acceleration. Even if you start slowly, you will find that you quickly reach your maximum speed. Learn to dig out that extra effort to find the additional speed within yourself—it is a great reward to find the extra speed that has been hiding from you.

CH. 9

## Follow-the-Wacky-Leader Fartleks

The running blahs descend on all of us from time to time. They may come from a long period of intense training for a particular goal, or a recent bout of

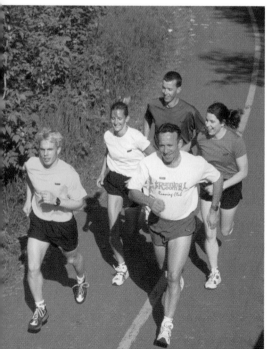

inclement weather can set you off. The best way to rid yourself of the blahs is to get some fun back in your running. I have used this fun drill with my running clubs over the years when things seem to be getting too serious.

First, call out a number as you point to each runner to number everyone in the group—it doesn't matter whether there are just two runners or a large group. Head out on your run, starting with 5 minutes of easy running to keep the group together. In order, each runner must decide on a fun fartlek or drill that the rest of the group has to participate in. Each drill should be 5 to 10 minutes long. Here are a couple of suggestions to get you started:

**Park Bench Jump:** Run a loop of about 150 metres and jump over a park bench. Hands are permitted.

**Beast Hill Workout:** My long-time training partner Mike O'Dell started this one when he spotted a killer hill of 150 metres with what looked like a grade of 60 percent. The rules call for only one hill repeat. No crawling is allowed and cheering is compulsory for everyone who reaches the top.

# Speed Training

Speed training is the roof of your training house. It is high-quality training that should only be done if you have spent adequate time in the strength and endurance phases of your training.

Speed training isn't for everyone. If you are a beginning runner or first-time marathoner, or if a time goal is not your priority, then continuing to work on your continuous or long run fitness with will be the most important aspect of your training. If you are looking for more specific results in an event, however, speed training can be an important phase in your preparation for the event. The principle of training specificity states that what a person does in their training will directly affect how they do in their races. Generally, this means that if you want to run an 8-minute mile (5-minute kilometre) in your event, you'd better get your body used to running at that pace in training. We break our speed sessions into shorter versions of the race, called intervals, that enable us to train at race pace.

CH. 9

## Pacing

Pacing is a critical aspect of successful speed training, because the goal is to maintain the desired pace for the entire workout—to finish each interval in the same amount of time. If you burn out and slow the pace during the last intervals, you probably started too fast; if you speed up throughout the workout, you probably started too slowly. Try not to become discouraged; pacing really takes practice.

Speed training uses short interval distances because the pace is hard enough that it can only be maintained for a short period of time (3 to 6 minutes). To keep your pacing simple, use your target race paces for the 1 mile, 5-K and 10-K. Be sure your goals are realistic. For example, don't choose a pace that would improve your 10-K time by 5 or 10 minutes. Work on improving your race times by no more than a couple of minutes at a time, no matter what the distance.

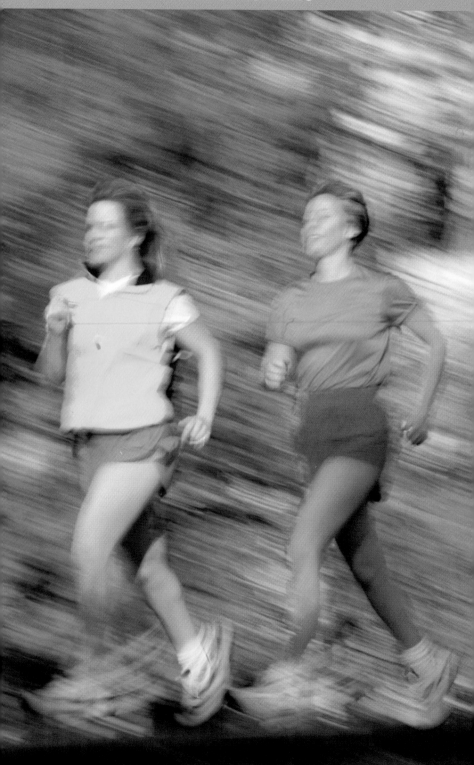

## Interval Distances

The nice thing about speed training is that the total distance covered during the workout isn't the most important aspect. Speed work intervals should be no longer than 1 mile (1.6 km) and no shorter than 400 metres. Use faster paces for the shorter distances and slower paces for the longer distances. For most runners, three to five intervals of a moderate length is a good place too start. To increase the total distance of your workout, make your intervals longer, rather than just increasing the number of repetitions. Add no more than 500 to 1000 metres of speed work each week.

## Rest Intervals

The rest intervals of your workout are a very important aspect of speed training. A good rule of thumb is to rest for as long is it takes you to run the interval. If it takes you 1 minute to run 400 metres, then rest for 1 minute before starting your next speed interval. Try to remain active during the rest interval. Walk or jog slowly; stopping or bending over to rest will delay your recovery and promote feelings of nausea or light-headedness. You can adjust the length of your rest period depending on your pace or how you feel. Remember, too much rest can defeat the purpose of the speed work and too little can poop you out before any training can be accomplished.

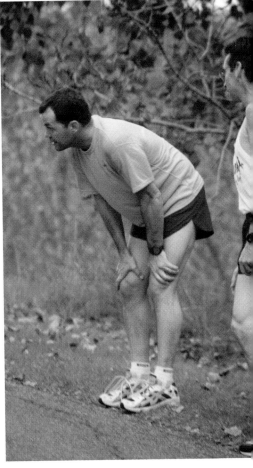

## The Speed Training Session

There are three components of a speed training session, and all three are critical to this type of training's success.

**Warm-up:** As discussed in chapter 5 (Stretching), a proper warm-up is crucial for any workout, but especially for speed training—the fast pace puts a lot of stress on your running muscles. Your warm-up should consist of at least 10 minutes of light aerobic activity (slow running) followed by 5 minutes of pre-stretching. A pre-stretch doesn't require you to hold the stretches for as long a period. In addition, you may want to cut down on the number of stretches you do and really focus on the working muscles of the legs and lower back.

**The Workout:** Plan, plan, plan. Always know what you are going to do before you get to the track or the start of a run.

**Cool-down:** A proper cool-down is important after a speed workout because your muscles have been working at a much higher intensity that usual. Your cool-down should always include at least a couple of miles of easy jogging or light aerobic activity (slow running) and stretching.

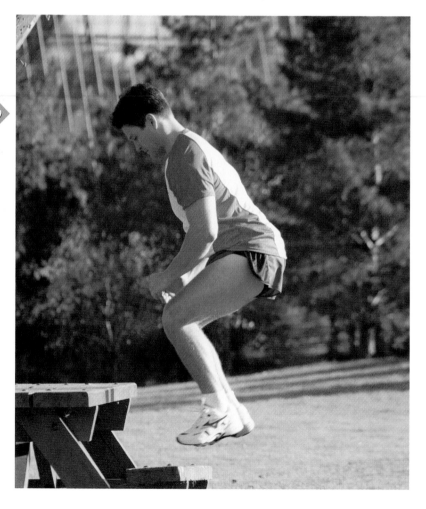

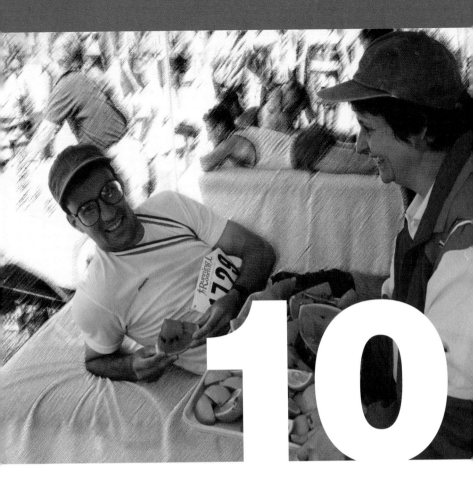

# 10 Nutrition

There are literally volumes of books dedicated to the topics of nutrition and weight control. A single chapter can only brush the surface of our understanding of nutrition, but the following pages should help provide you with appropriate guidelines to make healthy eating part of an active lifestyle.

A major issue facing most of us is how to make better choices in our daily intake of food and liquids. Think of one glass of water filled with your daily intake of calories and another glass filled with your daily output of calories through exercise and daily living. Simple enough. If you are at the perfect weight and body fat content, then you will strive to have the same amount of water in both glasses. For the vast majority of us trying to lose a few pounds, however, the goal is to have a larger glass for the output than for the input. (In reality, most of us enjoy more input than output.)

Many people become obsessed with the fat and oil contents of their food while neglecting to take note of the total number of calories consumed. Too many calories taken in, even from healthy foods like salads, breads and lean meats, still get converted to fat for storage, which is why exercise is so vital. The most important thing is a balance between the amount of exercise we get and the amount of food we consume. Intelligent choices in our food selections are what can really give us an advantage in weight management. More importantly, we must think of our total well-being rather than just the management of our body weight.

## The Scale

Do yourself a favour today and give your scale away, preferably to someone you don't like. A scale is one of the most useless things for us to use in managing our health. For the most part, it is only an accurate measure of how much water we have consumed and whether or not we are well hydrated.

Rather than using a scale to chart your progress, take some measurements of your chest, arms, thighs, calves, hips and waist. Mark them down and re-visit the measurements every couple of months.

An even simpler way to see your body change is to get a tight pair of pants, one that you can just barely stuff yourself into, and mark them. Those pants will be your benchmark of fitness today and into the future. Once a week, try on the pants to see how they fit.

Alternately, for those of you who are brave and not particularly concerned about modesty, stand naked in front of a mirror. What you see today is the start point. Once a week, make your trip to the full-length mirror. I do suggest that this be done alone; the mirror can be blatantly honest, and this is not the time for critics.

# Nutrition Basics

Most of us have read and heard enough about nutrition that we understand the basic functions of carbohydrates, fats, proteins, vitamins, minerals and water. For this book, we will focus on the role of nutrition in your training program. Think of food as fuel for your athletic body. The three main sources of fuel are carbohydrates, proteins and fats.

## Carbohydrates

Carbohydrates are the best source of energy for exercise, and they should make up 55 to 65 percent of your total energy intake.

There are two basic types of carbohydrates: simple and complex. Simple carbohydrates, such as those found in table sugar and fruits, are absorbed quickly into the bloodstream. In large quantities, these carbohydrates can give you a sugar high followed by a sugar low. The sugar high can provide quick energy, but the low is associated with feelings of lethargy and sometimes even nausea. Complex carbohydrates, which are found in foods such as pasta, potatoes, cereals and breads, are slower to be absorbed by the body; they provide the body with a slower, more steady stream of energy.

Once digested, carbohydrates are utilized in the body in the common form of glucose. Excess glucose can be stored in the muscles and the liver in the form of glycogen. When your carbohydrate intake exceeds your energy demands, carbohydrates can be converted to fat and stored in the fat tissues of the body. In men, fat traditionally collects first around the midsection; in women, around the hips. (Nature's sense of humour seems to be at work here, because that is also the first place we want the fat to leave.)

CH. 1

glucose

## Proteins

Proteins are the building blocks of the human body, and to meet your daily requirements they should make up 10 to 15 percent of your total calorie intake.

Proteins are made up of smaller units called amino acids—there are 20 different ones. When your body is in need of regeneration or repair, such as after running, amino acids provide the necessary materials. Your body can manufacture some amino acids, called non-essential amino acids, but you must obtain the others, called essential amino acids, through the foods you eat.

Food proteins that contain all the essential amino acids are known as complete

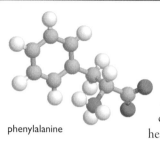

phenylalanine

proteins. Animal products, such as meat, eggs and milk products, are a great source of complete proteins. Animal proteins tend to be higher in saturated fat and cholesterol, however, so they should be eaten with some discretion. Choose lean cuts of meat and low-fat dairy products as part of a healthy diet.

In contrast, proteins that are missing one or more of the essential amino acids are know as incomplete proteins. Cereals, legumes and nuts contain incomplete proteins. Appropriate combinations of incomplete proteins, however, can provide adequate quantities of all the essential amino acids. If you are a vegetarian, you may want to consult a registered dietitian for a complete evaluation of your protein intake.

Most North Americans eat protein in excess, and excess amino acids that are not needed for regeneration or repair can become an energy source after the amino portion of the molecule is removed and excreted as urea. If your protein intake exceeds both your regenerative and energy needs, the proteins can be converted into fat for storage.

## Fats

**CH. 10**

Much has been written in recent years about the evils of too much fat in our diets. We need to eat fat, but it should account for less than 30 percent of your daily calorie intake, and you should be selective about the kinds of fat you eat.

There are two basic types of fats, saturated and unsaturated. Saturated fats are found in animal products, such as cheese, butter, meat and poultry, and some plant sources, such as palm oil, coconut oil and cocoa butter, and many of them are solid at room temperature. Unsaturated fats, which are found in plants and some fish, can be either monounsaturated or polyunsaturated. Monounsaturated fats are found in olive, canola and peanut oils and in avocados; polyunsaturated fats are found in safflower and sunflower oils and in salmon, tuna and sardines.

Too much fat, especially saturated fat, can contribute to higher levels of cholesterol, which is often feared because of its link to cardiovascular disease. What many people are unaware of, however, is that small amounts of cholesterol are essential to many functions in the body. Cholesterol is produced by the body as well as consumed in the diet, especially from animal products such as eggs, organ meats and shrimp. For people who are concerned about their cholesterol levels, it makes sense to lower their overall fat intake and pay attention to their cholesterol intake.

# Vitamins and Minerals

Vitamins are organic molecules that play a key role in many metabolic and cellular functions. They cannot be made in adequate quantities by your body, so you must acquire them through your diet. Unfortunately, there is no way to judge your vitamin levels unless you exhibit the symptoms of a deficiency or an excess of a particular vitamin. The best way to ensure that you have an appropriate amount of vitamins is to eat a healthy, balanced diet.

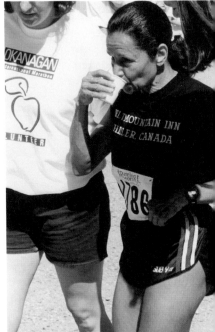

riboflavin

Minerals are inorganic elements that are also important for cell function, and they provide the building blocks for bones and teeth. As with vitamins, appropriate amounts of minerals can be obtained by eating a well-balanced diet. Most minerals serve many different functions: calcium is best-known for its role in bone formation, but it is also essential for the normal functioning of nerves and muscles; iron is a component of hemoglobin, which transports oxygen in the blood, and it is also needed for energy metabolism in cells.

Some people find that taking a multivitamin and mineral supplement is an easy way to ensure that they are meeting all their daily requirements. A better way is to eat a balanced diet following the national guidelines or, better still, consult a registered dietitian to have an assessment.

CH. 10

# Water

Drink water. When in doubt, drink more water.

The human body is made up of more than 60 percent water, and water is essential for many of our bodies' basic activities—blood is primarily water, and the perspiration that drives our body's cooling system is, of course, almost entirely water.

The sports medicine folks tell us that we need to drink 8 to 10 glasses of water a day to replenish our supply. We lose about 2 quarts (2 *l*) of fluid naturally each day; runners and other atheletes lose even more through exercise. Don't wait until you are thirsty; monitor your daily intake and take water with you on every run. There are some fine torso-packs that allow you to carry the water comfortably for any distance. Your training performance and recovery will improve through adequate water intake.

## Nutrition Basics

**Smart nutrition is variety, moderation and wholesomeness.**

**Water**
- **Drink 8 to 10 glasses a day, on top of what you drink during exercise.**
- **Carry a water bottle with you on all your runs.**
- **Drink during your winter runs, as well as during summer.**
- **Eat foods high in water (e.g., fruits, vegetables).**
- **Drink before you are thirsty.**
- **Drink water with all your meals.**

**Carbohydrates**
- **Eat carbohydrates daily to avoid depleting the glycogen in your muscles.**
- **Consume carbohydrates shortly after you exercise.**
- **Eat 8 servings of grains, fruits or vegetables each day.**

**Protein and Fat**
- **Eat proteins and fats in moderation.**
- **Think of carbohydrates as the main part of your meal and proteins as the condiments.**
- **Choose lean meats trimmed of excess fat.**
- **Avoid deep-fried foods and high-fat sauces when dining out.**
- **In fast food restaurants, choose salads without the dressing.**

**Iron**
- **Eat iron-rich foods, such as red meats, legumes, dark green vegetables, breads and cereals.**
- **Have your doctor do regular blood work to check your iron levels.**
- **Watch for signs of fatigue.**
- **Take an iron supplement if you are prone to anemia.**

# Energy Metabolism

Most people do not really care about a scientific analysis of the various energy systems, but a simple understanding of them will help you to train and fuel yourself in a more intelligent manner.

Carbohydrates, proteins and fats do not provide an immediate source of energy for our exercise; instead, they are used to manufacture a compound called adenosine triphosphate (ATP), an energy-rich substance that is stored in our cells. ATP can be created by different energy-liberating systems in the body, depending on the demands of the situation or exercise.

## Anaerobic Alactic System

If you run a short, all-out burst of 50 metres or do one maximal vertical jump, the energy comes from ATP that is already stored in your muscle cells. Only small amounts of ATP can be stored in the muscles and liver, so this energy-liberating system can only be used for a short period of time.

## Anaerobic Lactic System

If you run a fast 400-metre or 800-metre interval, a high-intensity activity that lasts for only 1 to 3 minutes, you use up your stored ATP and then produce more ATP through the breakdown of carbohydrates into lactic acid, which is a much more complex chemical reaction than the alactic system. More energy is supplied with the lactic system, but the by-product, lactic acid, is eventually responsible for the failure of the system when it accumulates to high levels. The lactic system is used during high-intensity training workouts like hill repeats and speed intervals.

CH. 10

ATP

## Aerobic System

If you are running for more than 3 minutes, you have to use the aerobic system, which can supply a large amount of energy over an extended period of time. The aerobic system uses oxygen to produce ATP through the breakdown of carbohydrates and fats into carbon dioxide and water.

Glycogen, the form in which carbohydrates are stored in the muscles, provides 60 to 70 percent of the fuel for the aerobic system during the first 20 minutes of exercise. If you continue to exercise for more than 20 minutes, fat becomes the predominate fuel source. Carbohydrates are the limiting factor in the fatigue of this system, and their depletion activates key chemical reactions used to liberate energy from fat.

If your muscle glycogen is fully depleted, the ability of the aerobic system to liberate energy from other carbohydrates and fats becomes severely limited and exercise will cease—commonly called "hitting the wall." The intensity and duration of the run, your diet and your current fitness level are all factors that affect the contributions of fats and carbohydrates to the total energy supply. Long slow runs train your body to use abundant fuel sources like fat more efficiently so you can exercise for longer periods. In addition, energy bars, gels and drinks can provide fuel for the aerobic system and spare glycogen so that exercise can continue on long runs.

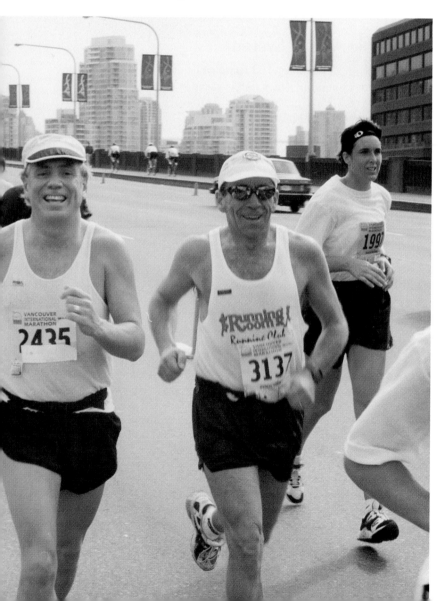

# Strength Training

## Strengthening Exercises

While stretching helps reduce your risk of injury by keeping tissues from becoming rigid and inflexible, strengthening can help prevent injuries by keeping weak muscles from being overpowered by stronger ones. There are three main opposing muscle groups involved in running that can be balanced by specific exercises:

Abdominals vs. Lower back

Quadriceps vs. Hamstrings

Shin vs. Calf.

Your hamstrings, for example, are vulnerable to strains if they are overpowered by your quadriceps. The hamstrings, therefore, demand both stretching and strengthening in a total conditioning program. Most people already have strong quadriceps, but these muscles can also benefit from further strengthening, which can prevent many overuse problems involving the kneecap. The lower leg can benefit from exercises that will improve its strength, balance, coordination and flexibility, which will result in a lowering of injury rates.

CH. 11

The following strengthening exercises should be done after you run, rather than before, or on a day when you are not running. They can be done three or four times a week.

## Foot Exercises

Why train the foot? Well, the longitudinal rib and the cross rib of the foot take a great deal of punishment during running, particularly during the landing and push-off phases. The ligaments and the aponeurosis plantaris that directly support the two ribs are passive tissues that cannot be trained; instead, the muscles of the foot can and must be trained in order to reduce the risk of injury. Your feet do a great deal of work for you during running, so give them some special attention each day and watch your strength improve over time.

Start with this simple exercise: drop a towel on the floor, stand with one foot on the towel and one off, and try to pick up the towel with your toes. After several weeks, proceed to this next exercise, which will strengthen your foot muscles, toe joints, ankles and knees: stand in a bucket filled with sand or rice and squeeze the sand or rice with your toes for 10 minutes.

## Ankle Exercises

Your ankle acts as a powerful lever during running. Over time, runners develop powerful running-specific muscles, but they sometimes neglect the development of improved coordination. Spend some time on these two drills and not only will they help improve your base running but they may help prevent a turned ankle on one of your runs.

*The Flamingo*

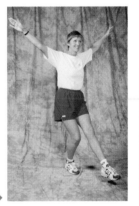

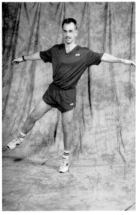

Start by balancing on one leg for 30 seconds without touching down with the other leg. When this balance becomes easy, try it with your eyes closed. You will notice it's much harder to hold a balanced position without visual cues. After mastering the blind flamingo, try bending your raised leg slightly at the knee and then do some toe raises.

Over the years I have spent a fair amount of time in airport line-ups, and I have found the flamingo to be the ideal exercise—not only do you get some interesting looks, but you must be careful not to lose your space in the line while your eyes are closed. (By the way, while the flamingo does require the one-legged stand, the pink tights are optional.)

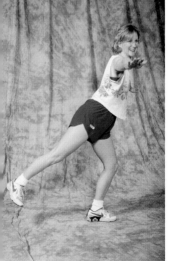

CH. 11

*Balance Kicks*

This drill can be done on a flat surface, or, to increase the complexity, try it on a rebounder. Stand on one leg, kick your other leg back, balance and hold for 20 to 30 seconds. Switch legs and repeat.

Repeat the exercise with kicks out to the side and in front of you. These positions will seem awkward when you first try them, but over time, as your balance improves, they will become more fluid—you may even think of signing up with the Dallas cheerleading squad.

## Push-ups

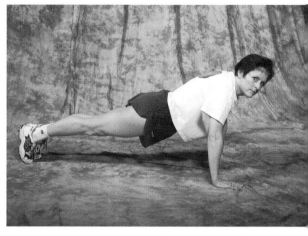

Yes, I am sorry to break the news to you, but your old phys-ed teacher was right: push-ups are good for you. Push-ups work on all the upper body muscle groups, improving your running form and posture. We all know how to do them; it's getting around to doing them that's a problem. This single exercise could replace a lot of time in the weight room if only we didn't find it so boring. Check off a daily 25 or so. Be sure to keep your back straight.

## Sit-ups (the right way)

CH. 11

We have all seen the many infomercials on the benefits of the latest abdominal equipment on the market. Well, save yourself a few bucks; do these sit-ups as part of your daily routine and those abs of steel will be yours! The great benefit of this sit-up is it works all the abdominal muscles from the rib cage through to the groin area. You, too, could have that infomercial "six-pack belly."

Lie flat on your back with your knees bent and your feet flat on the floor. Be sure to do an abdominal tuck to flatten the small of your back against the floor. Now extend your arms to put your hands on your thighs and then curl up your upper body, sliding your fingertips up to your knees. Keep the small of your back on the floor. Hold for a count of 10 and then lower yourself back to the floor. Start with about 25 repetitions and build from there.

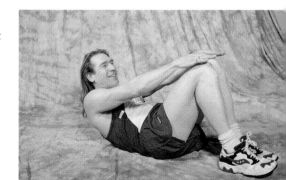

## Step-ups

Find a sturdy bench you can step on that isn't too high (your knee shouldn't bend tighter than 90 degrees when your foot is on the bench). Step up onto the bench and stand up straight before you step down. Alternate your feet each time. This drill works the upper leg muscles and hip flexors.

## Calf Raises

Stand on the edge of a step with your heels hanging over so that your toes carry your weight. Slowly raise and lower yourself. Start with both feet and then try one foot at a time. You can add a light weight after a few weeks of single-leg raises. This drill improves the strength and flexibility of the lower leg muscle group.

CH. 11

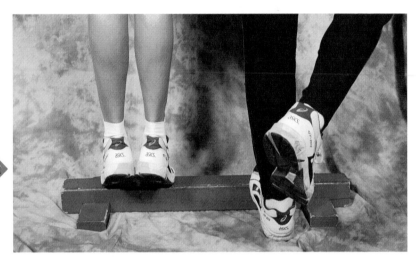

## Benefits of Strength Training

- **Helps reduce the risk of injury.**

- **Prepares your muscles for faster running.**

- **Makes you stronger on hills.**

- **Enhances the rehabilitation of skeletal and muscular injuries.**

# Weight Training

You are a runner, so it is important that your weight program is tailored specifically for your running requirements—you want to develop greater muscular endurance in your legs, arms, lower back and abdomen. Muscular endurance is the ability of a muscle or group of muscles to perform repeated contractions against a light load; training for muscular endurance will allow you to improve your strength without gaining the muscular bulk of a body builder. (The body builder shape may have some appeal on the beach, but you are using this program to enhance your running.)

The important thing to focus on in your weight routine is building endurance strength. Work out with weights that are fairly light—no more than 70 percent of the maximum weight you can lift—and work on doing more repetitions: three sets of 12 to 20 repetitions, with no more than 1 minute of rest between sets. Abdominal exercises should be done in sets of 30 to 50 repetitions.

Begin your program with a couple of weeks of even lighter weights so you can learn and practise good weight training form. To maintain flexibility, be sure to concentrate on performing a full range of motion; your movements should be smooth, fluid and controlled. Start with fewer repetitions and work your way up to 20 over several sessions. Once you have accomplished three sets of 20, it is time to increase the weight or resistance. With each change in weight, be sure to start with fewer repetitions and go through the same building process.

The following basic exercises, which work a large number of muscles, belong in every strength building program.

CH. 11

## Leg Press

Lie with your feet shoulder-width apart and your toes pointed slightly outwards. In the start position, your leg should be bent at 90 degrees. Push up until your legs are straight, but not locked. Lower to the starting position.

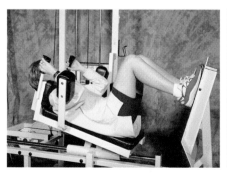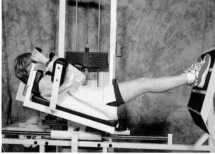

## Runner's Reach

Hold a dumbbell in each hand and stand with your feet shoulder-width apart. Now pump your arms in a running motion for a couple of minutes.

This exercise looks easy, but it is a fast and efficient way to tone up the old upper body, which will help you maintain good running form as you tire in the latter stages of a run. The postural muscle groups—the back, shoulder and abdominal muscles that control your posture—get the full benefit of this workout.

CH. 11

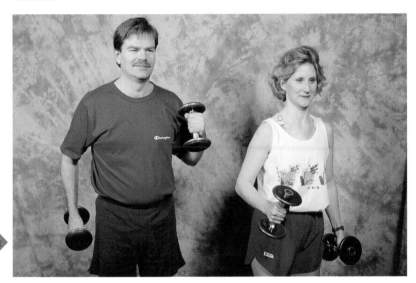

## Bench Press

Lie on your back on a bench. I prefer to have my knees up and my heels on the edge of the bench to force me to do a pelvic tilt, which keeps my abdominal muscles tight and my back flat against the bench. Lift either hand weights or a weight bar straight up from your chest until your arms are straight. Do not let the weight drift over your head or down to your stomach, and do not arch your back. Lower the weight slowly to your chest. This exercise can also be done on many weight machines.

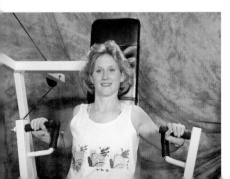
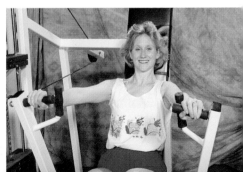

## Behind the Neck Press

Stand or sit up straight on a bench. Start with the bar behind your neck at shoulder height. Press it directly up over your head. Lower it slowly to the starting position.

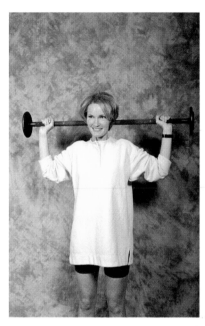 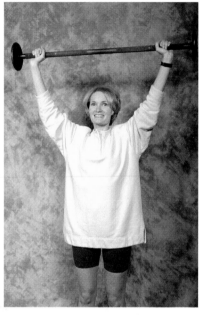

CH. 11

## Arm Curls

Stand or sit with your back straight, your head up and your feet slightly spread. Grasp the bar in an underhand grip. Start with your arms fully extended, slowly curl the bar up to your chest and then lower it to the starting position. Be careful to lower the weight slowly and to keep the movement under control.

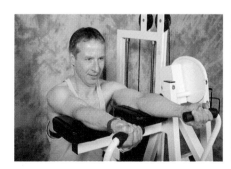 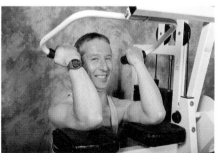

## Inclined Press

Lie against an inclined back rest. Start with the weight at your chest, with your arms at 90 degrees. Fully extend your arms in a controlled movement. Return the weight to your chest.

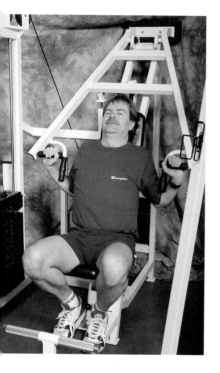
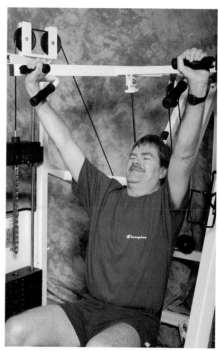

## Leg Extensions

Sit with the small of the back firmly flattened into the seat back. Extend and contract first one leg and then the other.

The most common error made with this exercise is to extend both legs at once; if you extend one leg at a time, you will discover any strength imbalances between your legs. By working each leg with the same amount of weight, you can eventually eliminate the imbalance.

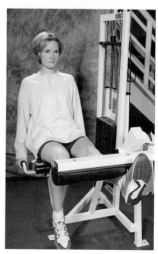

## Leg Curls

Lie on your stomach with the rollers on your calves and your knees off the bench. Curl up one leg as far as you can and then lower it until your legs are straight. Repeat using the other leg. If you exercise one leg at a time, it will keep you balanced.

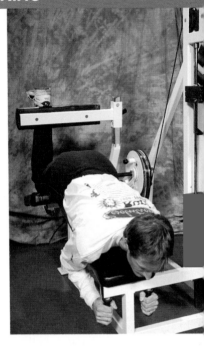

## RULES TO REMEMBER

- Perform your strength exercises two or three times a week.

- Sit-ups and push-ups can be done five times a week.

- Warm up with some easy running or biking before you start your weights.

- Give yourself at least **48** hours between weight workouts or a high-intensity run.

- The hard/easy system—load and rest, load and rest—will make you stronger.

CH. 11

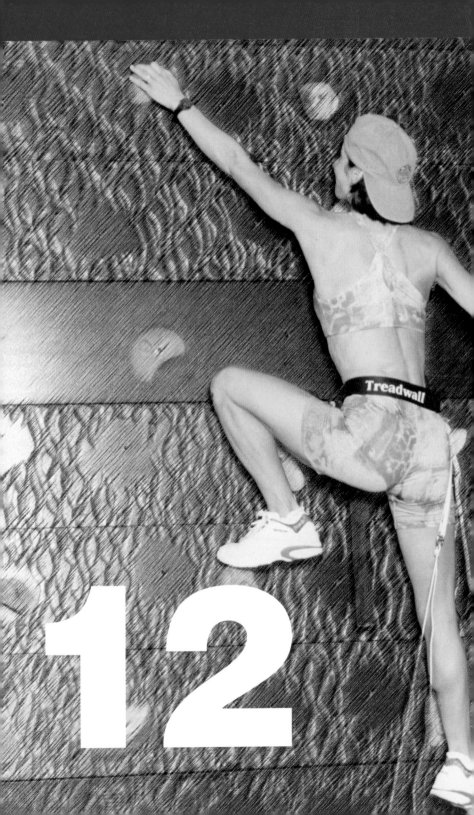

12

# Cross-Training

## How It Works

Cross-training is the practice of using two or more sports to enhance your overall fitness. *How will swimming improve my running?* some skeptics might ask. Simply put, by adding sports like swimming, cross-country skiing or aerobics to your running schedule, you can enhance your overall strength and cardiovascular fitness, and that can't help but improve your running performance. It is really very easy to explain, but first you need to know a bit about your body's adaptations to training.

Generally, through exercise training we make our bodies more efficient at delivering oxygen to the muscles and we make our muscles stronger. All aerobic exercise of sufficient intensity and duration will promote adaptations in both these categories: central adaptations improve the cardiovascular system (the heart, lungs and blood); peripheral adaptations improve the muscular system. The central adaptations in the heart, lungs and blood will carry over directly from sport to sport, but the location of the peripheral adaptations varies from activity to activity. Running predominantly requires the use of the legs, so most of the peripheral adaptations will be in the legs; swimming, on the other hand, mostly requires the arms.

CH. 12

Back to your question, *How will swimming improve my running?* Like running, swimming is a super aerobic activity, and when it is done at sufficient intensity and duration, it will improve the efficiency of your cardiovascular system, which will directly improve your running. Most of the muscular adaptations of swimming don't carry over to running, but you will be promoting whole body fitness, which is healthier in the long run than just focusing on the strength and efficiency of your legs.

The best cross-training regimens use a wide variety of activities that stress different muscle groups, which allows one muscle group time to rest and repair while you work on another group. Swimming and running are the best examples because they exercise such different muscle groups. Avoid activities that are too similar, because the predominant muscle groups may not get enough rest, resulting in fatigue or injury.

Another advantage of cross-training is that by combining weight-bearing and non-weight-bearing activities—running and swimming, running and cycling, running and rowing—you can give your joints a chance to rest and repair from the constant stress of weight-bearing activities.

## Cross-training Benefits

- **Enhance the quality of your training so you can receive maximum results in minimum time.**

- **Reduce your risk of injury.**

- **Add variety to your workout schedule.**

- **Help you stay fit even when you are injured or sore.**

- **Strengthen individual muscles and increase your overall strength.**

- **Promote smooth action between muscle groups.**

- **Improve your endurance levels.**

# Three Great Aerobic Sports

CH. 12

## Cycling

Whether you opt for a sleek 10-speed or a sturdy 15-speed all-terrain model, cycling can have many benefits that cross over to running:

- Balanced muscle strength between your quadriceps and hamstrings.

- More flexibility in your hips and knees.

- Improved hill running.

- Faster leg speed.

- Better cardiovascular endurance.

- Lower race times in events lasting more than 2 hours.

If you haven't ridden a bike since grade school, you may find your first outing fairly taxing, especially on your hands, buttocks, shoulders, neck and leg

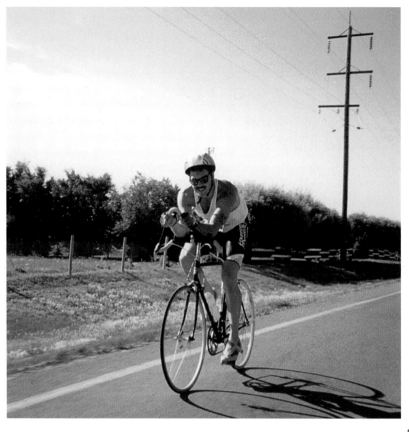

**CH. 12**

muscles. Be sure to get a bike that fits you—your muscles, joints and cardio-vascular system will thank you.

Obviously, the most sensible and enjoyable start to a cycling program is a slow one. If you run five or six days a week, begin by substituting bike rides on one or two of those days. Start with only 5 to 10 miles (8 to 16 km) of riding; you'll soon find yourself able to ride 20 miles (32 km) in a little over an hour on a flat course. For fitness purposes, 4 miles (6 km) of cycling is roughly equivalent to 1 mile (1.6 km) of running.

## Swimming

Swimming is a sport that cushions your muscles and gives you a great workout, to boot. By adding a swim to your weekly workout schedule, you can boost your aerobic fitness, upper-body strength, muscular endurance and breath control. If you spend about the same amount of time swimming as you would running, you'll get a roughly equivalent workout.

If you're not already an experienced swimmer, your first strokes in the pool may be a little difficult—your best approach is to wet your feet gradually. A good first goal might be just to swim one lap of a 25-metre pool. Eventually, you'll want to build up to swimming 1 mile (72 laps in a 25-metre pool) without stopping. Time isn't a factor in the beginning, but you should work steadily to increase your speed. Use the freestyle (front crawl) stroke to get the best overall workout.

## Cross-country Skiing

Cross-country skiing does more than just replace the pounding and jarring of running with a kick and glide that's gentle on your legs; it works the large muscles of your arms, torso and back, as well as your leg muscles, to provide an unparalleled cardiovascular workout.

As with any other new activity, it's best to start slowly and build your mileage as you become more accomplished. For the easiest start, head to a nordic centre that sets tracks on its trails. The tracks will keep you moving along in a straight line so you can concentrate on your form without worrying about the terrain.

Even for the beginner, cross-country skiing requires some special equipment—skis, boots, bindings, poles and light but warm clothing—so you'd be wise to rent it the first few times just to make certain that you like the sport. Once you're sure, consult a seasoned skier and inquire at several shops to get skis, poles and bindings that match your size and ability.

### What about resistance training?

**Cross-training works best when two or more aerobic activities are combined throughout the week. Weight or resistance training gives cross-training a bit of a twist because it promotes whole-body improvements in strength, but not cardiovascular fitness. Weight training won't lead to vast improvements in your running performance, but the benefits of moderate weight training a couple of times a week are substantial—having stronger muscles and tendons and balanced joints will help decrease your chance of injury and will help you tone up the spots that your aerobic activities might miss. (See chapter 11 [Strength Training].)**

# Water Running

## Benefits of a Water Workout

Water running allows you to follow the same action as running on land, using water as the resistance, but without the forces of impact on the bones and soft tissues of the legs. It was originally developed for injured athletes, because the cool water and the low impact of the workout allow runners to maintain their all-important cardiovascular systems while they recover from an injury. Additionally, the extra resistance of the water builds stronger muscles, joints and tendons, which helps prevent future running injuries. Running in the water is such an efficient exercise that many injured athletes have jumped out of the pool and run personal best times after not having run on land for up to a month.

Over the years, many runners who first tried water running when they were injured discovered that they could use it to recover from hard training sessions while still getting in a workout. There has been enough written about stress, rest and the benefits of a hard/easy training program that we all appreciate the importance of rest, and water running has now become part of the regular training regimes of beginners and elite performance runners alike.

Your heart rate will be lower during a water workout because of the buoyancy and the cooling effect of the water, so you are able to get a great cardiovascular workout without the pounding and risk of injury. Stay relaxed and enjoy the massage benefits of water running: your knees, ankles and joints will all be stronger and suppler after a period of water training.

One of the major reasons many runners take up water running is for the social aspects of a group run. Because your forward motion is not an important measure intensity in water running, a very wide range of talents can run together—a 6-minute-miler and a 9-minute-miler can go work out together, carrying on a conversation and keeping each other company, unlike on dry land.

CH. 12

Beginning runners can benefit immensely from water running because its low impact gives some much-needed stress relief to a body that is used to a sedentary lifestyle. The new runner's muscles, ligaments and joints are supported by the cool water while they burn extra calories through the advantage of double resistance—the faster you run in the water, the more the resistance. Water running is a safe, controlled environment in which a novice runner can try out running.

Average runners may find that hopping into the pool on a weekly basis is a good way to improve their flexibility; in the water, they can do running drills to improve their range of motion that they would not be able to do on dry land. One especially effective drill is to perform a bounding run, much like a sprinter in slow motion: kick your forward leg out far in front of you and maintain a high back kick as you bring your other leg around. All runners can use water running to work on their form. In the water, all of your actions are accentuated because of the slow-motion effect, so it's an excellent time to do a form check on your running.

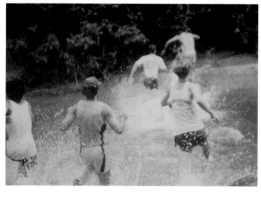

Pregnant women can find it easier to exercise throughout their term, thanks to the positive effects of water running: they benefit from the cooling effect of the water, they avoid undue muscular stress and their heart rates stay lower. In addition to the usual advantages of exercise, a fit woman can experience a shorter recovery time following delivery. Water running is an excellent alternative that a pregnant woman should discuss with her physician. For more information, see chapter 13 (Women's Running).

Elite, high-performance runners can use water running to intensify their workouts far above normal levels. An elite runner who suspects an injury is imminent can take a rest from the pounding of road running and break up the normal training schedule with a water run. Older runners, too, may find that the low impact of water running allows them to work out more often than they could if they were only running on land. Many athletes who at one time did two runs a day are now doing the second workout in the water—they add more mileage to get more speed with less injury risk.

**CH. 12**

## How to Do It

OK, now it is time for you to hop into the water and experience a whole new form of running. The pool should be deep enough that you can't touch bottom without submerging your head. Wear a water vest that will keep you floating at about shoulder level and help you maintain an upright running position. I know of some runners who are able to water run without a vest, but in the interest of maintaining good running form, I recommend that you use one— many public pools have water vests available for you to use or rent.

Start your workout with a normal running motion. Focus on your form, keeping your shoulders back, bringing your knees up high, and tucking your ankles under your buttocks. To keep your arms in the correct motion and in tune with your leg movements, you will find that you have to concentrate on driving your elbows back with each motion. Keep the motion of your arms forward and back—think of a sprinter running and keep your hands slicing through the water. Don't let your arms cross your body and don't do any sculling actions with your arms or hands. Keep your sprinter's form to avoid spinning rather than running—spinning will give you a good fat-burning workout, but by keeping your proper form, you can work on an improved range of motion. The effects on your running form of this slow-motion workout will become apparent after only a couple of sessions.

Here are is a sample, high-performance workout that should keep your interest up and your boredom level down:

• Warm up with some deep-water jumping jacks.

• Swim with the water vest on, doing some gentle breaststroke moves.

• Float on your back and pull your knees up to your chest several times for a modified sit-up drill.

• Focus on your form for 10 minutes of easy running.

• Do a 30-second sprint followed by 30 seconds of easy running. Repeat once.

• Do a 45-second sprint followed by 30 seconds of easy running. Repeat three times.

• Do a 1-minute sprint followed by 30 seconds of easy running. Repeat three times.

• Do a 45-second sprint followed by 30 seconds of easy running. Repeat three times.

• Do a 30-second sprint followed by 30 seconds of easy running. Repeat once.

• Cool down with 10 minutes of gentle running.

CH. 12

Another way to break up your workout if you find the time dragging is to count the number of leg turnovers you have each minute or each lap.

The exercise value of a workout in the water is very close to that of running on dry land, so spend about the same time in the water as it would take you to run the targeted distance for that day. For example, if you are scheduled to run an easy 7 miles (11 km) and your pace for easy running is about 8 minutes a mile (5 minutes a kilometre), go for a 56-minute water run.

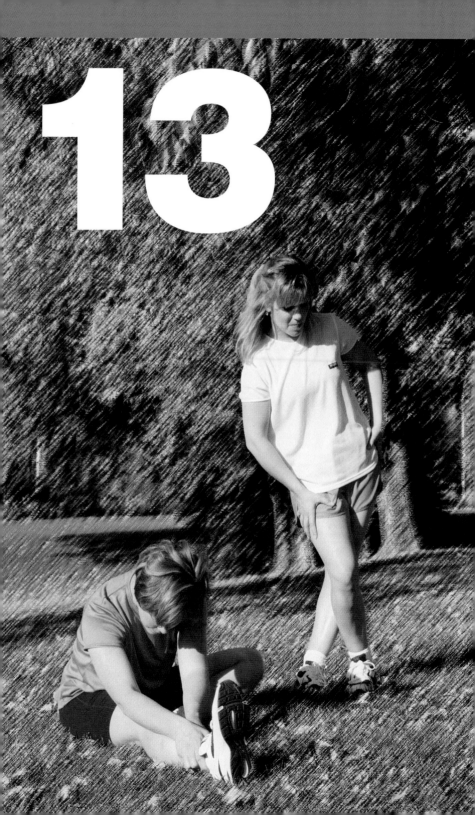

13

# Women's Running

Everyone needs regular exercise to stay healthy: for both men and women, it offers weight loss, reduced levels of harmful cholesterol, fewer sick days and improved self-esteem. Weight-bearing exercises build and maintain strong bones in both sexes, and people who exercise have fewer headaches and less lower back pain, anxiety, depression and fatigue. Women can also experience some special benefits from running: certain menstrual symptoms, including appetite changes, breast tenderness, fluid retention and mood changes, may be eased; and the stronger bones that develop through weight-bearing exercise may help prevent osteoporosis after menopause.

## General Health Issues

There are many physiological differences between men and women—women tend to have smaller hearts, less lung capacity, smaller muscles and more body fat—and, in particular, women often have questions about how exercise relates to their menstrual cycle and reproduction. By answering their questions and learning how to avoid possible pitfalls, women can enjoy the benefits of a full exercise program.

## Hormonal Changes

For some women, especially those with little body fat, too much exercise can reduce the levels of the hormones estrogen and progesterone, which control menstruation and help bone growth. The reasons for exercise-related hormone changes are complex and not well understood. What is known, however, is that these changes can be reversed with small reductions in training or small weight gains.

The menstrual effects of low hormone levels can range from normal periods with no egg production, to infrequent or light periods (oligomenorrhea) to no periods at all (amenorrhea). For girls near puberty, the onset of menstruation may be delayed by intense exercise. Changes in the menstrual cycle can have an effect on fertility, but this usually only occurs with excessive training. Certainly, women who have irregular periods, no matter what the cause, should see a doctor.

If hormone levels are low for a long time, such as during too much exercise, calcium will be lost from the bones. This loss is similar to that which occurs after menopause, and it can result in more easily broken bones, especially the spine and hips. Women who have a history of irregular periods should have their bone density measured to determine if there has been any associated bone loss. More often, however, the skeletal adaptations to weight-bearing exercise will improve a woman's bone density.

## Risk of Injury

A question that is often asked about women in sport is whether they are at higher risk of injury than men. This concern, which has no basis in fact, kept women from taking part in many sports until recently. For example, women were not allowed to compete in the Olympic marathon until 1984.

The body's response to exercise is the same for both sexes. Each sport puts its own demands on the body and carries its own risk of injuries, and women are at no greater risk of these injuries than men. The important thing is for a training

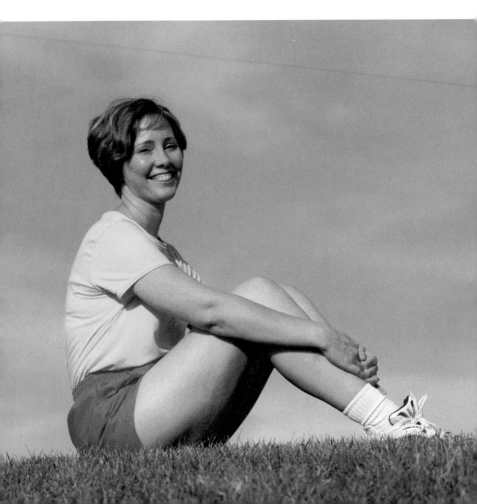

program to be suited to the individual's fitness level, regardless of their sex. Any sports injury should be treated promptly by a doctor.

## Iron Levels

All athletes must maintain proper iron levels in their bodies. Iron is a key element in hemoglobin, the compound that carries oxygen in the red blood cells, and it is also an important part of many body proteins and cell components.

Women who menstruate risk having low iron levels because of their monthly loss of blood (and therefore iron). Very active women have an added risk, because high-intensity exercise can impair the absorption of iron by the gastrointestinal system. They also lose iron in their sweat and experience a breakdown of red blood cells in some of the tissues.

All women should eat a diet with enough iron. Red meat is the best source of iron. Any red meat and the dark meat of poultry provide a form of iron called heme-iron, which is more easily used by our bodies than the iron found in vegetables and grains. The most effective way to get enough iron is to combine red meats with vegetable proteins. For example, split pea soup with ham and chicken soup with lentils are high-iron combinations. Vitamin C, which is plentiful in fruits, will increase your iron absorption. Calcium, on the other hand will hinder your iron absorption, so it's a good idea to pass up that glass of milk with red meat and have it with toast or cereal instead.

Some people who restrict meat from their diets are also counting calories, and in the process they may cut back on other food groups that supply iron. One way to increase your iron intake, especially if you are limiting calories, is to choose breads, cereals and pastas with added iron—they usually say "enriched" or "fortified" on the label.

The single or combined effect of iron loss through menstruation, exercise and diet restrictions can cause an iron deficiency. The symptoms of low iron include tiring easily and poor athletic performance. If your iron stores become too low, you can develop anemia, which has the added symptoms of paleness, greater fatigue and shortness of breath. Women should have their hemoglobin levels checked by a doctor on a regular basis. For those at risk of low iron, the body's iron stores should also be measured.

CH. 13

## Good Sources of Iron

| Meat | Iron (mg) per 4-oz. (113-g) serving |
|---|---|
| Pork chop | 4.6 |
| Sirloin steak | 3.9 |
| Turkey (dark meat) | 2.7 |
| Lamb (leg) | 2.5 |
| Lean ground beef | 2.4 |
| Chicken | 1.3 |
| Tuna | 1.3 |

| Fruits, grains & vegetables | Iron (mg) per $1/_2$-cup (113 ml) serving |
|---|---|
| Dried apricots | 6 |
| Dates | 5 |
| Baked beans | 3 |
| Kidney beans | 3 |
| Raisins | 2 |
| Spinach | 2 |
| Green beans | 1 |
| Enriched pasta | 1 |

# Calcium Needs: A Matter of Age

Proper calcium intake is one of the keys to fighting osteoporosis, a disease in which the bones become thin and porous. What that proper amount is, however, depends on a woman's age.

Most women's skeletons stop growing at around age 17. During the preceding

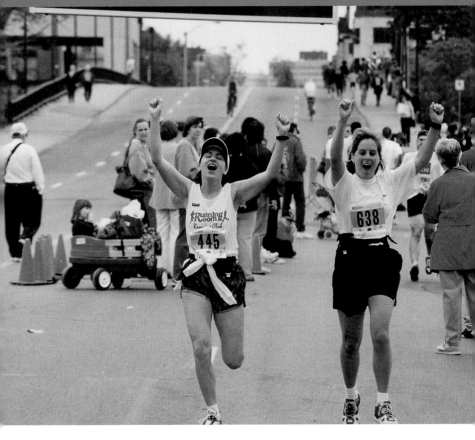

building period, 1200 mg of calcium are needed daily to assure maximum growth. Although the skeleton has stopped growing after that, the bone density can increase by as much as 10 percent up to around age 30 to 35, so continuing to get 1200 mg of calcium a day is probably your best bet. Reaching the maximum bone density during these years is critical, because if a greater mass of bones is developed in youth, there is less danger of osteoporosis when they inevitably start to thin with age.

Once the peak bone density is reached, the years before menopause appear to be a holding period. The minimum daily calcium intake to maintain bone density during these years is 800 to 1200 mg. Amounts beyond this minimum don't seem to carry an extra benefit, and women athletes who are not menstruating will lose more bone mass than average, even if they have a high calcium intake.

After menopause begins, bone density will be lost. Unfortunately, high calcium intake seems to have little or no effect in early post-menopausal years—the apparent futility of slowing bone loss at this time makes good habits earlier all the more important.

Does all this information suggest that popping calcium supplements throughout life is key to preventing osteoporosis? Calcium supplements can help some people, but eating a well-balanced diet is really the best way to obtain the right quantities of vitamins and minerals.

# Exercise and Pregnancy

## Benefits

The benefits of maintaining your exercise program through your pregnancy are not well documented, but that shouldn't detract from your own perceptions of your program; the advantages of exercise training in general may help prepare women for the physical and psychological stresses of pregnancy and labour.

Exercise not only increases aerobic capacity, it also increases insulin sensitivity in the muscles, which means the body can mobilize and oxidize fat more quickly, decreasing the race of glycogen depletion during exercise. Improved muscular strength may help in maintaining a feeling of agility, and it may be especially beneficial in carrying added weight and dealing with a change in the centre of gravity, which moves lower and forward during the course of pregnancy, thereby preventing back pain. A few scientific investigations have even reported that women who maintained their fitness during pregnancy had elevated levels of B-endorphin during labour and delivery, thereby reducing their pain perception.

## Safe Running Quiz

Safety questions to ask during your pregnancy (and at any other time).

- Is the area appropriate for the exercise activity?
- Is it relatively safe and free from latent defects and danger?
- Is it free from rapid and changing environmental conditions?
- Is it relatively safe from criminal activity?
- Is it well populated?
- Is it close to emergency facilities?
- Is it close to telephones?

## Commonly Reported Benefits

- **Maintained aerobic capacity.**

- **Increased insulin sensitivity.**

- **Improved muscular strength.**

- **Decreased pain perception.**

- **Positive well-being.**

- **Self-acceptance.**

## General Concerns

Care must be taken when you exercise during pregnancy, because both exercise and pregnancy put stress on the body, particularly on the back, hips, knees and other joints and muscles. If you are already active, you can probably continue to exercise if you modify your program as the pregnancy advances and pay attention to how you feel and what your doctor recommends. The planning and implementation of your exercise regimen should be under the strict supervision of your doctor. Consult your doctor before you even begin. A woman, especially during pregnancy, has to make sure she has good pelvic floor and abdominal muscle support before beginning a running program.

The physiological and anatomical changes in a woman's body during pregnancy are generally considered to inhibit exercise. It is not known whether or not the anatomical changes that occur, such as the loosening of the joints and ligaments, together with the increased weight and the continuing shift in the centre of gravity, mean that pregnant women have a greater risk of strains and sprains than the general population. The extent of the body's adjustment to these changes depends on many factors, both external and internal. Individual factors, such as age, body weight and health status, are significant, as well as the type of exercise undertaken and the environment in which it is performed.

CH. 13

Little is known about the effects on a fetus of the mother's exercise, but pregnant women should certainly avoid contact sports to reduce the risk of injury to the abdomen. They should also lower the intensity of activities such as racquet sports and some field games to reduce the risk of injuries.

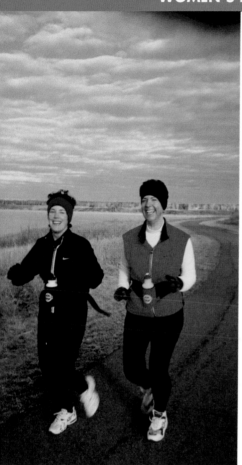

# Running and Walking

Women who were not running before their pregnancy should not take it up until after delivery—combining the stresses of pregnancy and an unaccustomed exercise would invite injury or complications. If you have already been running, however, you can safely continue your program throughout your pregnancy as long as you take certain precautions.

During the first trimester, women should be aware that certain common complications, including nausea, vomiting or poor weight gain, can affect their running programs. Even without these complications, women should shorten their running distances to no more than 2 miles (3 km) a day to reduce the risk of hyperthermia (over-heating) and dehydration. Because pregnant women are running to maintain fitness, rather than training for competition, the

**CH. 13**

shorter distances should suffice. If you want to exceed these recommendations, you should coordinate it with your physician to allow for closer follow-up.

During the second and third trimesters, the increase in a woman's body weight may make running more difficult, and other factors, such as lower limb swelling, varicose veins and joint loosening, may also affect performance. In particular, because the joints loosen in preparation for delivery, pregnant women need to be especially careful to run on an even path.

Because of the nausea and general feeling of fatigue that many pregnant women experience, however, you may not be able to run long distances. Also, be aware that ketosis (increased fat metabolism) and hypoglycemia (low blood sugar) are more likely to occur during prolonged strenuous exercise in pregnancy.

Walking is always a more-than-reasonable alternative to running, especially if running becomes uncomfortable as the pregnancy progresses. A walking program could consist of 4- to 6-mile (6- to 10-km) walks, depending on the terrain and temperature. The same precautions should be taken in preventing dehydration and hyperthermia.

The buddy system is a must for pregnant women, particularly when you exercising outside in the extreme cold, where there is a potential for hypothermia. Remember, fitness is more fun with family or friends.

## Pregnancy Exercise Guidelines

- **Do not begin a running program while you are pregnant.**
- **Do not exercise if it is hot and humid (above 100° F [38° C]).**
- **Wear walking or running shoes with proper support.**

## Water Running and Aquasize

Water running is a great way to relieve the stresses of normal running, and the difference in cardiovascular benefits is minimal. Pregnant women benefit from the cooling effect of the water, which helps keep the body's core temperature at normal levels and the heart rate lower.

Water running is usually done in deep water with the help of a flotation device to keep you above the surface and in an upright position (see p. 137). Flotation devices are often uncomfortable for pregnant women, however, so the workout is moved to shoulder-deep water.

You should be trying to simulate the running action as much as possible. Don't lean too far forwards. Keep your shoulders back and bring your knees up high, tucking your ankles under your buttocks and you perform your strides. Your arms should move in time with your legs, swinging naturally against the water for an upper-body workout. For variety, stride sideways, backwards and forwards. You may even want to try some aerobic dance steps. Begin with 15 to 30 minutes in the pool, depending on your fitness level.

CH. 13

Water running and aquasize (water exercise) are most fun done in groups. Check with your local community pool or fitness facility for a convenient aquasize program.

## Avoiding Hyperthermia (Over-heating)

**If you live in a warm climate or need to exercise and there's no alternative to working out in hot weather, there are a number of precautions you can take:**

- **Acclimatize gradually to the temperature.**

- **Avoid the worst of the heat by exercising early in the morning or in an air-conditioned facility.**

- **Wear clothing that will permit the free evaporation of sweat.**

- **Drink plenty of fluids.**

- **Do not exercise when you are ill.**

- **The buddy system works well to monitor heat distress.**

## Running Through Pregnancy

### by Sandy Bellan

When I got pregnant, I'd been running for nearly four years, and I knew that I didn't want to give it up. Running was fun, it provided great stress relief, and it was a part of my routine. As all regular exercisers know, your workout sometimes seems like the only constant in a hectic and changing life, and since I knew my body and my life were going to change dramatically, I was quite determined to keep this constant in place!

CH. 13

I knew that since I was already active, I could safely continue with moderate exercise throughout my pregnancy. The problem, however, was that I wasn't interested in exercising moderately; I wanted to continue what I was doing.

My first thought was that since my body was already used to a certain level of activity, I should be able to just carry on as usual. I wanted to be sure that it was safe, however, so I started to look through running books, exercise books and pregnancy books to see what I could and couldn't continue to do.

What I found was that there was very little specific information on how safe it was to run through pregnancy, and most of the advice was aimed at women who were sedentary. Even the running books offered only general guidelines. Many of them cautioned against getting too hot, especially in the first trimester. While this turned out to be one of the most important pieces of advice I followed, I found myself wondering, What exactly is too hot? While I knew that racing would probably be out, I wondered if going for a long run would make me too hot, or even running a short distance on a hot day.

Here are some practical tips that made me feel safe when I ran:

- Eliminate your weekly long runs. I knew that the longer I ran, the more heat I would produce. Some conservative guidelines suggested limiting runs to 20 minutes. While I didn't want to cut my runs that short, I knew hour-and-a-half runs were out!

- Use a heart rate monitor. I always kept my heart rate at around 75 percent of my maximum, which for me was around 145 beats a minute. If the monitor showed I was going over this, I just backed off.

- Drink even more water than usual before your runs.

- Keep your body temperature below 100° F (38° C). In the first trimester, I took my temperature immediately after running a few times, which was very reassuring. My temperature was always below 98.6° F (37° C) even after a run on a very hot day. I knew from then on that even when I felt quite hot, it didn't mean my body temperature was soaring up.

- Take your pulse 5 minutes after the workout to make sure your heart rate has dropped below 100 beats a minute. This recovery consistently happened for me and showed that I wasn't pushing myself too hard.

- Run with a partner. During the pregnancy I made sure I always ran with my regular running partner. It proved to be quite a sacrifice on her part, because our outings gradually turned from running to near walking!

CH. 13

- Reduce your weekly mileage and the frequency of your runs. When I got pregnant I immediately decreased the length and intensity of my runs in order to avoid over-heating. I still kept the weekday runs at about 45 minutes, but I eliminated the long runs.

- Run progressively less often and less far as the pregnancy progresses. In my first trimester, I was still averaging roughly 12 miles (19 km) a week and feeling very fit and healthy. Because the physical aspects of pregnancy hadn't begun to slow me down, the hardest part at this stage was making myself run slower. In the second trimester, my increasingly different size and shape began to limit my running sessions. For me, at least, it seemed to happen quite suddenly, and even though I averaged about 7 1/2 miles (12 km) a week over this trimester, there was a dramatic difference in the length and intensity of my runs from the beginning of this period to the end.

- Expect changes in your heart rate. In the first weeks of the second trimester, I was still pretty much carrying on as usual, but then an interesting physio-logical change started to happen: even when I was running the same route at my usual pace, my heart rate began to soar. My heart was having to work harder to let me run at the same pace, which signalled the beginning of slowing down.

I stopped running at around 8½ months, because the pounding was just too uncomfortable. I didn't want to give up the stress relief that running provided, however, so I switched to other aerobic exercises: I went to the gym and rode a stationary bike or used the stair climber or the rowing machine. Despite some strange looks, I continued with this routine until two weeks before my daughter was born.

I know that my experience wouldn't be right for every pregnant woman. I know that some women are too sick or too tired in the first trimester to keep up their old routines, and, obviously, if you're having complications and your doctor advises you not to run, then don't. Pregnancy is short in the big scheme of things; you've got your whole life to run. We all have different pregnancies and different limits. Near the end of my pregnancy, I knew when I was ready to stop running. If you run during your pregnancy, you'll recognize that point, too.

The jury is still out on whether being fit decreases the length or intensity of your labour, but I can tell you from my experience that being fit helps you tolerate the stresses of labour better, and it absolutely helps you to recover faster afterwards.

So what happened at the end of this journey? I got a very healthy and rather large daughter. We're still running together, except now she's in the baby jogger, where she seems to feel right at home.

**CH. 13**

## Pregnancy and Later Fitness

### by Kathy Morgan

At the onset of my first pregnancy, I made a decision to stop the exercise program I had followed for many years. My program had comprised running twice a week and swimming or aerobics twice a week. My blood iron level was significantly lower than it should have been, despite the fact I was taking the maximum dosage of an iron supplement. At four months, I had gained no weight and my doctor told me that if my iron level did not increase he would be giving me a blood transfusion. I decided I was not going to have a transfusion so I found out what foods were high in iron. I began to eat Cream of Wheat for breakfast and other foods fortified with iron. My blood iron level did not worsen so I did not have to have a blood transfusion. I was so concerned about this aspect of my health that I did not ask my doctor about the benefits or ill effects of exercise during pregnancy.

I gained 32 pounds in total during the pregnancy and gave birth to my daughter, who weighed 8 pounds, 9 ounces. I joined aerobics classes when my daughter was six weeks old, and it took me six months to get to my pre-pregnancy weight.

When I got pregnant the second time, I felt great. I had no morning sickness, no problem with my blood iron level and I gained weight at a steady pace. I joined a prenatal aerobics class and went twice a week. The instructor was a wonderful lady. She had us running laps, doing sit-ups and monitored every participant to ensure we were exercising correctly. I went until I was eight months pregnant. I kept up with all the exercises, but I found that any movements that involved stepping sideways made me feel sick—I had to turn myself and face the direction I was going.

I gained 25 pounds during this pregnancy and gave birth to my son, who weighed 7 pounds, 12 ounces. Immediately after the delivery, my stomach went very flat. The attending nurse was kneading my stomach and said to the student nurse, "This one has good stomach muscles." When my son was 10 days old I could fit into most of my clothes.

I cannot say whether exercising with one pregnancy made the delivery any easier, because both labours were about 12 hours in length and both times I had severe back pain. But, without question, I felt a million times better physically after my second pregnancy.

CH. 13

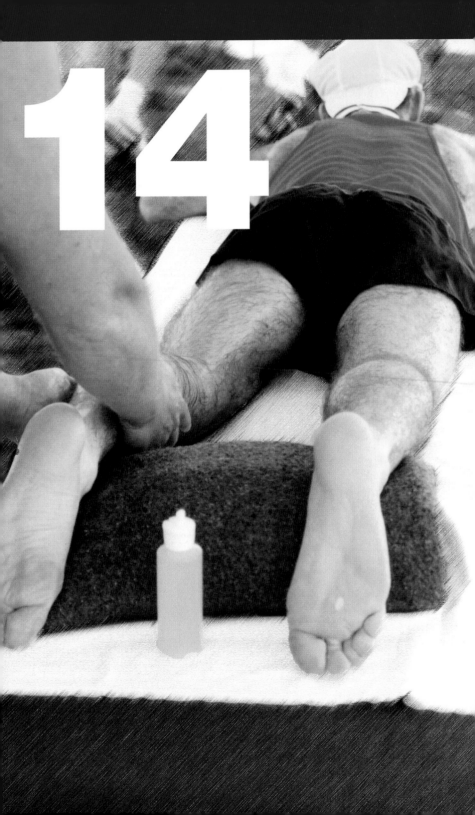

14

# Running Injuries

Most runners are highly motivated and extremely devoted to their sport—they think that if they don't get their run in, they won't feel quite right—but while they are in pursuit of those miles, many forget to listen to their bodies.

Avoiding injury is not impossible if you pay attention to your training techniques and don't try to do too much, too soon. The best way to prevent most athletic injuries is to maintain good muscle strength and flexibility.

Most running injuries are from overuse, so tune in to your body and listen to what it's telling you. If you're cranky or more impatient than usual, you may need a few days of rest. Other signs of fatigue are a susceptibility to colds or flu, difficulty falling asleep, an inability to sleep well, a higher than usual resting pulse rate or more than the usual aches and pains in the limbs. The one running maxim you should never forget is "any pain, no brain."

## Common Causes of Injury

- **Too many miles, too quickly.**
- **Running in improper or worn-out shoes.**
- **Insufficient rest, such as running too hard on "easy" days.**
- **Lack of a good mileage base.**
- **Forcing a run when you're tired.**
- **Pushing too hard during intervals and tempo runs.**
- **Too much speed training or too many hills.**

## Causes of Injury

Running injuries can be divided into two basic categories: those caused by an acute trauma and those resulting from overuse.

## Traumatic Injuries

Traumatic injuries are violent and sudden, such as sprains, lacerations, torn ligaments, pulled muscles or broken bones caused by a fall, and they usually require immediate professional treatment. If you hear or feel a crack, tear or pop and the pain persists, or if the injury causes swelling, an inability to use the injured body part or pain that does not subside in 30 to 40 minutes, you should seek immediate professional help.

## Overuse Injuries

Overuse injuries are more common than traumatic injuries, and they develop from mild or low-grade, repeated stress over a long period of time. The knees and the soft tissues of the lower leg are most susceptible to overuse injuries. Anatomical imperfections, such as flat or high-arched feet, an abnormally sized or positioned kneecap or inequal leg lengths, can cause overuse injuries, but more than half are caused by training errors. Each run stresses the body, and daily, high-intensity training will not give the body enough time to adjust and recover. An imbalance of hard and easy workouts can also contribute to overuse injuries.

The best way to avoid overuse injuries is to understand the effects of long-term exercise on the bones, joints and muscles. Use a conditioning program that includes stretching, strengthening exercises and cross-training, and make sure you take the time to select proper shoes and socks. For more information, see chapter 2 (Building Your Program) and chapter 3 (Shoes and Clothing).

# Basic Care of Athletic Injuries

The pain associated with overuse injuries is usually not severe—it is often ignored by athletes—and it is more difficult to determine whether or not an overuse injury needs professional attention. If the pain persists for more than 10 to 14 days after you follow basic self-care treatments, such as decreasing the level of activity, applying ice, taking aspirin or ibuprofen and stretching, you should seek professional help.

CH. 14

Each type of overuse injury has specific treatments, but there are some general rules that can be applied to all injuries:

- Follow the R.I.C.E regime (Rest, Ice, Compression, Elevation).
- Reduce the distance and intensity of your runs for 7 to 10 days.
- Re-evaluate your training habits.
- Never run through pain. If the pain is severe at the beginning of and during the activity, the activity should be stopped completely. If the pain is

present at the beginning of the activity, but lessens and does not return until a few hours later, then the level of activity should be reduced.

- Consider using other aerobic activities to maintain your cardiovascular fitness while you rest the injury.

- Reduce inflammation by icing the area after the activity and by taking aspirin or ibuprofen throughout the day.

- Encourage healing with a whirlpool, a massage or ice and heat therapy.

## The R.I.C.E. Treatment

**Rest: Avoid any activity that could make the injury worse.**

**Ice: The type of ice is not as important as making sure it is applied.**

**Compression: It is easiest to compress the injury with a stretch elastic bandage (tensor type), wrapping towards the heart.**

**Elevation: During and after the application of ice, the injured body part should be elevated above the level of the heart.**

**Do an initial assessment of the injured limb. Within 5 to 10 minutes following injury, apply an ice pack directly to the injured area, wrapping it firmly in place with a wide elastic wrap. Be sure to check that your circulation isn't impaired, and take care not to freeze the underlying tissue. Elevate the injury well above the level of your heart and leave the ice pack in place for 20 minutes. After removing the ice pack, reapply the elastic wrap for compression and continue to elevate the body part. Reapply ice every 2 hours during the first 48 hours, and do not use compression while you are sleeping.**

# Achilles Tendinitis

Achilles tendinitis, one of the more difficult injuries to treat in athletes, involves the inflammation, degeneration or rupture of the Achilles tendon. The Achilles tendon is located at the back of the heel, and it inserts into the rear portion of the heel bone.

## Symptoms

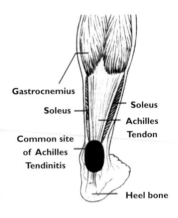

Gastrocnemius

Soleus

Soleus

Achilles Tendon

Common site of Achilles Tendinitis

Heel bone

The symptoms of Achilles tendinitis tend to come in stages or degrees of severity:

**Stage 1:** The runner experiences a burning or prickly pain in the Achilles tendon about 1 to 3 inches (3 to 8 cm) above the heel bone. The pain results from the inflammation of the vascular sheath that surrounds the tendon, and it may simply be due to irritation from the shoe.

**Stage 2:** The Achilles tendon itself becomes inflamed (tendinitis) and the pain becomes a shooting or piercing sensation that occurs during the activity, especially when you change direction or run uphill. It is common to feel more pain at the beginning and after the activity.

**Stage 3:** The collagen protein fibres in the tendon weaken to the point that the tendon will snap or rupture, causing a great deal of pain.

## Causes

The positioning of the Achilles tendon at the base of the calf makes it susceptible to running injuries, which can have many causes:

**CH. 14**

• overpronation, which strains the soleus muscle of the calf;

• supination or high arches, which strain the gastrocnemius muscle of the calf and cause injury high up in the Achilles tendon;

• constant rubbing of the back of the shoe against the tendon;

• improper shoe selection;

• inadequate warm-ups;

• direct trauma;

- dramatic increases in the period or intensity of exercise;

- heel bone deformity;

- high-mileage, long-term running programs that do not incorporate enough rest.

## Treatment

### Short-term

- Decrease the distance and intensity of your runs for 7 to 10 days.

- Never run through pain.

- Avoid hills.

- Treat the heel with ice after every run.

- Follow a flexibility program that concentrates on the calf muscles and includes stretching and heel lifts.

- Take aspirin or ibuprofen—never acetaminophen—to reduce the inflammation.

If the injury persists for more than two weeks, you should see a doctor.

### Long-term

To prevent Achilles tendinitis from recurring, or ever occurring, all runners should be aware of their personal shoe requirements. You should buy shoes that are designed to correct any gait problems you may have, such as overpronation or supination, and you should replace your shoes periodically as they deteriorate. A continuous flexibility program is also important. Some runners may need to seek professional help, either to get semi-rigid orthotic devices for their shoes, or, in extreme cases, to have the tendinitis treated directly by a doctor.

CH. 14

# Iliotibial Band Syndrome

Iliotibial band syndrome is one of the leading causes of lateral knee pain in runners. The iliotibial band is a superficial thickening of tissue on the outside of the thigh that extends from the outside of the pelvis to just below the knee. During a normal gait cycle, the iliotibial band moves from behind the femur to in front of it, and it is crucial to the stabilization of the knee. The continual rubbing of the band over the bone, combined with the repeated bending and

Quadriceps

Common site of Iliotibial Band Syndrome

Hamstring

Femur

Patella

Insetion of Iliotibial Tract

extension of the knee during running, may cause the area to become inflamed, or the band itself may become irritated.

## Symptoms

The symptoms of iliotibial band syndrome range from a stinging sensation on the outside of the leg just above the knee to pain along the entire length of the tissue at the point where the band moves over the femur. The pain may not occur immediately, but it will worsen during activity when the foot strikes the ground if you over-stride or run downhill, and it may persist afterwards.

## Causes

Iliotibial band syndrome can be caused by poor training habits or anatomical abnormalities:

- running on a banked surface, such as the shoulder of a road or an indoor track, which causes the downhill leg to bow outwards slightly and puts extreme tension on the band against the femur;

- inadequate warm-up or cool-down;

- running excessive distances or increasing your distance too quickly, especially if it is combined with running on a cambered surface;

- bow legs or tightness of the iliotibial band, which both put tension on the band against the femur.

## Treatment

### Short-term

Treat the functional problems resulting from poor training:

- Decrease your training distances.
- Ice the knee after activity.
- Alternate your running direction on a pitched surface.
- Stretch as much as the injury will allow.

### Long-term

To treat structural abnormalities, such as a natural tightness in the iliotibial band, you should employ a stretching program, especially before working out, to make the band more flexible and less susceptible to injury. In extreme cases, it is possible for surgery to relieve tightness in the band.

**CH. 14**

# Plantar Fasciitis

Plantar fasciitis is a persistent pain located on the bottom (plantar surface) of the heel. The plantar fascia is a fibrous, tendon-like structure that extends the entire length of the bottom of the foot, beginning at the heel bone and extending to the base of the toes. During excessive activity, the plantar fascia can experience continuous stress and excessive pulling, which cause irritation or inflammation and may even tear the plantar fascia. Forefoot or toe running can cause micro-tears of the plantar fascia at the heel.

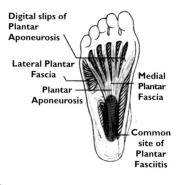

Digital slips of Plantar Aponeurosis

Lateral Plantar Fascia

Plantar Aponeurosis

Medial Plantar Fascia

Common site of Plantar Fasciitis

## Symptoms

The pain of plantar fasciitis is most noticeable with the first few steps in the morning, and it subsides with prolonged walking. Likewise, during athletic activity the pain will occur in the beginning of the exercise routine and subsides as the activity continues.

## Causes

Plantar fasciitis is more common in runners who have a high-arched, rigid type of foot or a flat, pronated foot. Improper shoe selection can also be a contributing factor.

- The most common cause is running on the forefoot or running up hills.

- In a high-arched foot, the plantar fascia is tight and band-like, causing it to be too rigid during the gait cycle.

- The plantar fascia is stretched by excessive motion in runners who overpronate.

- Improper shoe selection can cause excessive foot stress. Be sure to consider your foot and gait type when buying shoes.

- Stiff-soled shoes can cause stretching of the plantar fascia.

- Overworked shoes can allow the foot to pronate excessively.

**CH. 14**

## Treatment

To determine the proper treatment for plantar fasciitis, you must identify and eliminate the factors that caused the injury; a complete medical history and gait analysis are required.

## Short-term

- Ice application.

- Complete rest or a reduction in the intensity of exercise.

- Physical therapy involving whirlpool and ultrasound.

- Anti-inflammatory medication, such as pills or cortisone injections, to alleviate severe pain is considered a last resort for chronic cases only.

## Long-term

In persistent cases, orthotic devices can help correct biomechanical problems and alleviate stress and strain on the plantar fascia:

- High arches require softer orthotic devices for shock absorption.

- Flattened arches require a semi-rigid orthosis to control pronation.

To prevent the recurrence of the injury, exercises should be done to stretch the plantar fascia and the calf muscles. Most patients respond to these treatments, and only a very small percentage require surgery.

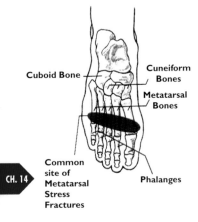

Cuboid Bone

Cuneiform Bones

Metatarsal Bones

CH. 14

Common site of Metatarsal Stress Fractures

Phalanges

# Stress Fractures

Stress fractures are tiny, incomplete breaks or cracks in a normal bone that are caused by repeated trauma or pounding. The crack occurs when the bone cells cannot rebuild as quickly as the repetitive trauma damages the bone. One of the most misdiagnosed of athletic injuries, stress fractures can happen after a short period of stress, but they more commonly result from a longer period of continued trauma. They can occur in both the upper and lower body, but they are most common in the foot.

## Symptoms

The pain of a stress fracture begins gradually and intensifies with continued activity. Pain is always present as an early warning, but it is often ignored by runners. Swelling and tenderness may also affect the area. One of a doctor's best methods to diagnose a stress fracture is if pain is felt when pressure is applied directly over the area. X-rays of the injured site should be taken, but the fracture may not show for up to 14 days after the injury. When stress fractures are ignored, the results can be serious—complete breaks in the bone, especially in the hip area, can mean surgery or prolonged disability.

## Causes

Most runners who suffer from stress fractures are in good physical condition and lack previous ailments that would have predisposed them to injury. Stress fractures are usually caused by poor training habits:

- switching to a harder running surface;
- a rapid increase in speed or distance;
- returning to intense activity after a layoff;
- inadequate rest;
- excessive stress;
- a change in footwear without a proper adjustment period;
- an improper shoe selection for the foot type.

## Treatment

### Short-term

- Rest—immediately discontinue the activity that caused the injury.
- Ice the injured area.
- Elevate the injury.

### Long-term

If the pain and swelling do not subside after a few days of self-prescribed care, and if athletic as well as normal activities become difficult, you should seek professional help:

- A cast may be used in tibial (lower leg) stress fractures.
- Metatarsal (foot) stress fractures may require casting for four to six weeks, because these bones are more difficult to immobilize.
- A heel cup or special protective padding can protect heel fractures.
- Crutches can relieve pressure and weight from the leg.
- Oral medications can alleviate pain and swelling.

The return to athletic activity should be delayed for as long as possible—from 4 to 26 weeks depending on the location and severity of the injury. The pain

CH. 14

may subside after the second week of treatment, but returning to a normal exercise routine can delay healing and cause permanent damage. Low-impact aerobic activities, such as swimming, rowing, cross-country skiing, walking or bicycling, can be used to maintain cardiovascular fitness.

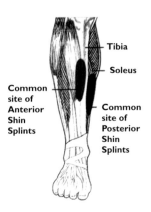

Tibia

Soleus

Common site of Anterior Shin Splints

Common site of Posterior Shin Splints

## Shin Splints

The lower leg pain of shin splints is caused by very small tears in the leg muscles at the point of attachment to the shin. Anterior shin splints occur on the front portion of the tibia (shinbone) and posterior shin splints occur on the inside (medial) part of the leg along the tibia.

## Symptoms

The pain may begin as a dull aching sensation after running. It can become more intense, even during walking, if it is ignored. Tender areas are often felt as one or more small bumps along either side of the tibia.

## Causes

Both anterior and posterior shin splints are caused by excessive stress being placed on the muscles of the lower leg, such as by overpronation, which overworks the muscles of the foot and leg as they try to stabilize the foot. Anterior shin splints are also caused by muscle imbalances, insufficient shock absorption and toe running:

- Tightness in the calf muscles, which propel the body forward, places additional strain on the anterior muscles of the lower leg, which work to lift the foot upwards and also prepare the foot to strike the running surface.

- Worn or improper shoes increase the stress on the anterior leg muscles. Softer surfaces and shoe cushioning materials absorb more shock so that less is transferred to the shins.

- Running only on the balls of the feet (toe running), without normal heel contact, puts a tremendous amount of stress on the lower leg muscles.

A rapid increase in the speed or distance of your runs can also overstress your lower legs. Remember: build your training program by no more than 10 percent a week (see p. 25).

# Treatment

## Short-term

As with most overuse injuries, a self-enforced treatment of shin splints is successful in most cases:

- Use aspirin or ibuprofen, never acetaminophen, to reduce inflammation and relieve pain.

- Ice the shin immediately after running—never before.

- Reduce your speed and distance for 7 to 10 days

- Never run through pain.

- Avoid hills and intense running.

- Use a varus wedge to support the inside of your foot and reduce pronation.

- Gently stretch your calf and thigh muscles.

## Long-term

Persistent shin problems may warrant a visit to a sports medicine specialist, who may prescribe the following treatments:

- strength and flexibility programs to correct muscle imbalances (to be done only in the absence of pain);

- orthotic devices;

- anti-inflammatory medications;

- physical therapy involving ice massage, ultrasound, electro-stimuli and heat to reduce inflammation and pain.

# Runner's Knee

Chondromalacia patella, "runner's knee," occurs when repeated stress on the knee causes inflammation and a gradual softening of the cartilage under the kneecap (patella). The inflammation of the cartilage prevents the kneecap from gliding smoothly within the femoral groove (a groove on the end of the thighbone). Runner's knee accounts for

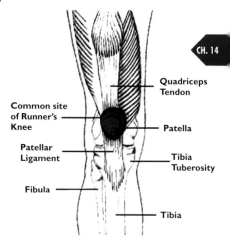

CH. 14

Quadriceps Tendon

Common site of Runner's Knee

Patella

Patellar Ligament

Tibia Tuberosity

Fibula

Tibia

25 percent of the overuse injuries treated in sports clinics, and any active person 14 or over may experience it.

## Symptoms

Runner's knee is typically associated with pain and swelling of the knee that increases gradually over a period of time, often a year or longer, until it is severe enough that the runner seeks medical attention. The symptoms usually occur beneath or on both sides of the kneecap, and the pain may be intensified by some activities, such as lunges, squatting or jumping. Stiffness may occur simply from prolonged sitting or descending stairs.

## Causes

The most common cause of runner's knee is overpronation, which rotates the lower leg inwards and causes the kneecap to move in an abnormal side-to-side motion instead of gliding within the normal track of the femoral groove. The tilt in road surfaces can accentuate foot pronation, so runners may experience pain in one knee if they continually run along the same side of the road.

Muscle imbalances can also lead to runner's knee. An imbalance of the quadriceps, in particular, may contribute to the injury, because the quadriceps normally aid in the proper tracking of the kneecap.

Repeated trauma, a history of previous trauma or an untreated ligament injury can also contribute to runner's knee.

## Treatment

### Short-term

- Decrease your training volume, and consider substituting swims. (When you are recovering, it is best to avoid any exercise that puts weight on a bent knee.)

- Rest if your knee is painful or swollen.

- Treat your knee with ice for 15 minutes twice daily and after the activity to reduce pain and inflammation.

- Take aspirin or ibuprofen, or consult your doctor about more sophisticated and effective anti-inflammatory medications.

### Long-term

Physiotherapy, including stretching and strengthening exercises for the quadriceps, hamstrings and calves, or orthotic devices to correct abnormal biomechanics

**CH. 14**

may be required in some cases. Once the causes are determined and the appropriate steps have been taken to treat the condition, runner's knee should not keep you from activity.

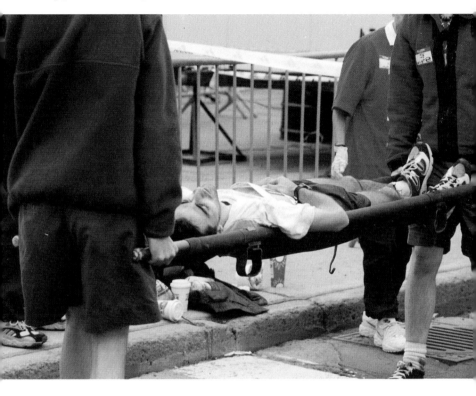

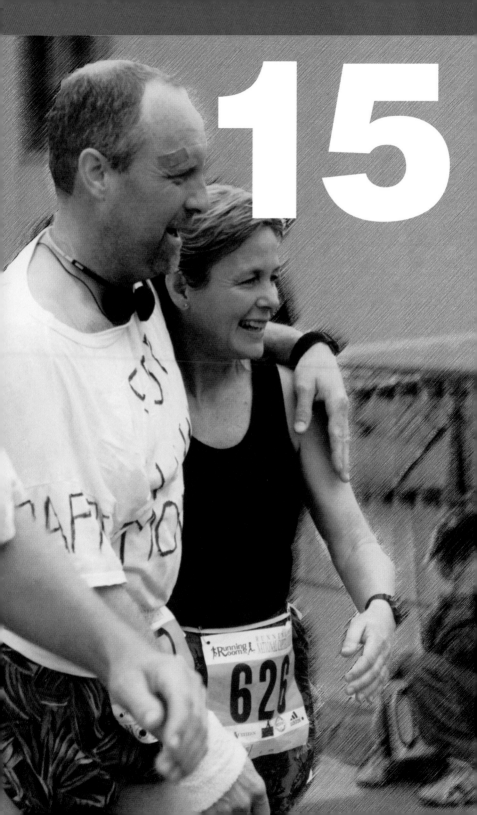

15

# The 10-K

The increasing popularity of the 10-K road race over the years comes from the fact that it requires only a limited amount of training, which can fit into most busy schedules, and you recover quickly after the race. For most of us, it is a fun event—you usually end up with a new T-shirt, great conversations with fellow runners, some food and a sense of accomplishment. The 10-K race can be a simple benchmark to judge your current fitness, or it can be a real test of athletic and competitive abilities, and the distance is short enough that most runners can enter the event with only simple modifications in their normal training.

You will find that running the occasional 10-K will add some spark to your running. It can also serve as a motivational force to get you out the door on those days when you really do not feel like running. The thought of running with a buddy in a weekend race will keep you out on those training runs during the week.

Most runners can comfortably run a 10-K every couple of weeks. Combining an intelligent training program that is in line with your current fitness level allows you to improve your running times. Sometimes, staying a couple of footsteps in front of a training buddy can be the motivating force to push you that extra little bit. If a time goal is not high on your priorities, then running

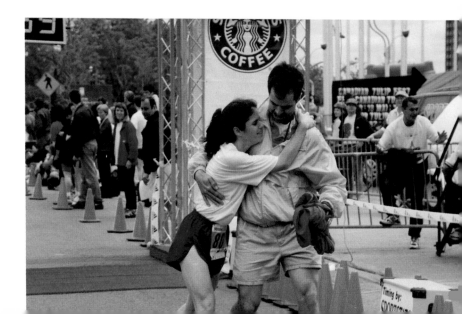

more comfortably and enjoying the race may be your goal. Keeping it fun and intelligent usually leads to satisfying results.

## 10-K Tune-up

Many runners find that when the local 10-K race season arrives they are left wondering how they can improve their race times when they just never seem to have time to go to the track for speed work. Here is a very simple workout that you can use once a week for eight weeks to sharpen your times for that 10-K season:

**Odd Weeks**

- Warm up with 10 to 15 minutes of easy running.

- Do some light strides to pick up the speed.

- Run for 4 minutes at a pace that is slightly faster than your current 10-K race pace.

- Recover with 5 minutes of easy running.

- Start with four intervals; add one interval a week; hold at a maximum of eight intervals.

**Even Weeks**

- Warm up with 10 to 15 minutes of easy running.

- Do some light strides to pick up the speed.

- Run for 8 minutes at your current 5-K race pace.

- Recover with 5 minutes of easy running.

- Start with two intervals; add one interval a week; hold at a maximum of five intervals.

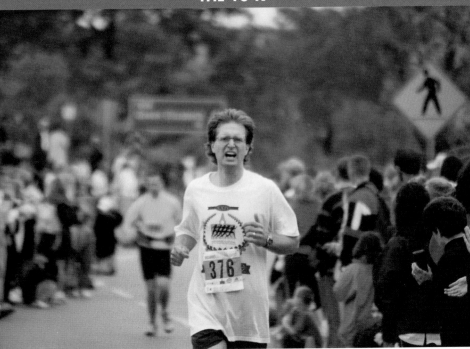

The training schedules on the following pages will help you prepare for a 10-K race. Choose the schedule that best reflects your targeted finish time. There are two schedules for each time goal: the first one presents the training distances in miles; the second in kilometres. A simple bar graph at the bottom of each page summarizes weekly changes in the distance of the long (Sunday) run and in the total weekly distance.

If you are running your very first 10-K, finishing in a smiling upright position should be foremost in your mind—smiling and upright makes for the best photos. For all runners, the best advice for the 10-K is to keep it fun! The more relaxed and focused you are at the start of the race, the more likely you are to achieve your goal for the race.

Going into your first 10-K, it is a great confidence builder if you have already run the distance. If you have not been able to achieve the distance in training, be sure to add in walking breaks of 1 minute for every 10 minutes of running.

**CH. 15**

If you have selected your parents well enough that you are able to run a 10-K in under 38 minutes (for which there is no schedule), follow the 80 percent rule: once you can run 80 percent of the race distance at your targeted race pace, you are ready to race the distance and achieve that target on race day. Start with once-a-week running sessions at race pace, progressively increasing the distance of these runs until you are running 80 percent of the race distance at your targeted race pace.

# To complete a 10-K
*training program*

*kilometres*

| | SUN | MON | TUES | WED | THURS | FRI | SAT |
|---|---|---|---|---|---|---|---|
| **Week 1** | off | off | 6 km<br>steady run | off | 5 km<br>steady run | off | 3 km<br>steady run |
| **Week 2** | 6 km<br>steady run | off | 6 km<br>steady run | off | 6 km<br>steady run | off | 3 km<br>steady run |
| **Week 3** | 6 km<br>steady run | off | 6 km<br>steady run | off | 6 km<br>steady run | off | 3 km<br>steady run |
| **Week 4** | 8 km<br>steady run | off | 6 km<br>steady run | 3 km<br>steady run | 6 km<br>steady run | off | 3 km<br>steady run |
| **Week 5** | 8 km<br>steady run | off | 6 km<br>steady run | 3 hills<br>85% effort<br>3 km warm-up<br>3 km cool-down | 6 km<br>steady run | 5 km<br>steady run | off |
| **Week 6** | 10 km<br>steady run | off | 6 km<br>steady run | 4 hills<br>85% effort<br>3 km warm-up<br>3 km cool-down | 5 km<br>steady run | 6 km<br>steady run | off |
| **Week 7** | 10 km<br>steady run | off | 8 km<br>steady run | 5 hills<br>85% effort<br>3 km warm-up<br>3 km cool-down | 5 km<br>steady run | off | 6 km<br>steady run |
| **Week 8** | 11 km<br>steady run | off | 6 km<br>steady run | 6 hills<br>85% effort<br>3 km warm-up<br>3 km cool-down | 8 km<br>steady run | 5 km<br>steady run | off |
| **Week 9** | 11 km<br>steady run | off | 8 km<br>steady run | 8 km<br>tempo run | 5 km<br>steady run | off | 6 km<br>steady run |
| **Week 10** | 13 km<br>steady run | off | 8 km<br>steady run | 5 km<br>tempo run | off | 3 km<br>race pace | off |
| **FINALE !** | 10 km<br>RACE DAY! | | | | | | |

- weekly total
- long run

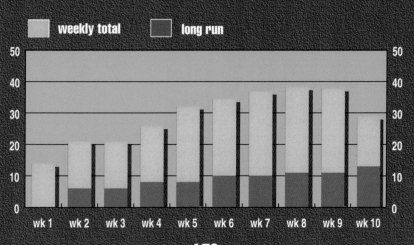

# To complete a 10-K
*training program*

*miles*

| | SUN | MON | TUES | WED | THURS | FRI | SAT |
|---|---|---|---|---|---|---|---|
| **Week 1** | off | off | 4 miles<br>steady run | off | 3 miles<br>steady run | off | 2 miles<br>steady run |
| **Week 2** | 4 miles<br>steady run | off | 4 miles<br>steady run | off | 4 miles<br>steady run | off | 2 miles<br>steady run |
| **Week 3** | 4 miles<br>steady run | off | 4 miles<br>steady run | off | 4 miles<br>steady run | off | 2 miles<br>steady run |
| **Week 4** | 5 miles<br>steady run | off | 4 miles<br>steady run | 2 miles<br>steady run | 4 miles<br>steady run | off | 2 miles<br>steady run |
| **Week 5** | 5 miles<br>steady run | off | 4 miles<br>steady run | 3 hills<br>85% effort<br>2 mi warm-up<br>2 mi cool-down | 4 miles<br>steady run | 3 miles<br>steady run | off |
| **Week 6** | 6 miles<br>steady run | off | 4 miles<br>steady run | 4 hills<br>85% effort<br>2 mi warm-up<br>2 mi cool-down | 3 miles<br>steady run | 4 miles<br>steady run | off |
| **Week 7** | 6 miles<br>steady run | off | 5 miles<br>steady run | 5 hills<br>85% effort<br>2 mi warm-up<br>2 mi cool-down | 3 miles<br>steady run | off | 4 miles<br>steady run |
| **Week 8** | 7 miles<br>steady run | off | 4 miles<br>steady run | 6 hills<br>85% effort<br>2 mi warm-up<br>2 mi cool-down | 5 miles<br>steady run | 3 miles<br>steady run | off |
| **Week 9** | 7 miles<br>steady run | off | 5 miles<br>steady run | 5 miles<br>tempo run | 3 miles<br>steady run | off | 4 miles<br>steady run |
| **Week 10** | 8 miles<br>steady run | off | 5 miles<br>steady run | 3 miles<br>tempo run | off | 2 miles<br>race pace | off |
| **FINALE !** | 6.2 miles<br>RACE DAY! | | | | | | |

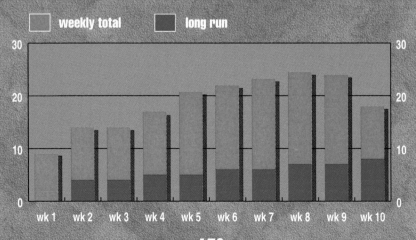

■ weekly total   ■ long run

173

# 55 minute 10-K
*training program*

*kilometres*

| | SUN | MON | TUES | WED | THURS | FRI | SAT |
|---|---|---|---|---|---|---|---|
| **Week 1** | off | off | **6 km** steady run 5:40 pace | **4 hills** 85% effort 3 km warm-up 3 km cool-down | **6 km** steady run 6:00 pace | **5 km** form/tempo 5:30–5:45 pace | off |
| **Week 2** | **6 km** steady run 6:20–6:30 pace | off | **6 km** steady run 5:40 pace | **5 hills** 85% effort 3 km warm-up 3 km cool-down | **6 km** steady run 6:00 pace | **5 km** steady run 5:30–5:45 pace | off |
| **Week 3** | **10 km** steady run 6:20–6:30 pace | off | **6 km** steady run 5:40 pace | **6 hills** 85% effort 3 km warm-up 3 km cool-down | **6 km** steady run 6:00 pace | **6 km** steady run 5:30–5:45 pace | off |
| **Week 4** | **10 km** steady run 6:20–6:30 pace | off | **6 km** steady run 5:40 pace | **7 hills** 85% effort 3 km warm-up 3 km cool-down | **6 km** steady run 6:00 pace | **6 km** steady run 5:30–5:45 pace | off |
| **Week 5** | **13 km** steady run 6:20–6:30 pace | off | **8 km** steady run 5:40 pace | **8 hills** 85% effort 3 km warm-up 3 km cool-down | **8 km** steady run 6:00 pace | **8 km** steady run 5:30–5:45 pace | off |
| **Week 6** | **16 km** steady run 6:20–6:30 pace | off | **8 km** steady run 5:40 pace | **9 hills** 85% effort 3 km warm-up 3 km cool-down | **8 km** steady run 6:00 pace | **8 km** steady run 5:30–5:45 pace | off |
| **Week 7** | **13 km** steady run 6:20–6:30 pace | off | **8 km** steady run 5:40 pace | **10 hills** 85% effort 3 km warm-up 3 km cool-down | **6 km** steady run 6:00 pace | **6 km** form run 5:30–5:45 pace | off |
| **Week 8** | **16 km** steady run 6:20–6:30 pace | off | **8 km** steady run 5:40 pace | **4 speed int.** 400 m in 2:00 3 km warm-up 3 km cool-down | **8 km** steady run 6:00 pace | **8 km** form run 5:30–5:45 pace | off |
| **Week 9** | **16 km** steady run 6:20–6:30 pace | off | **8 km** steady run 5:40 pace | **5 speed int.** 400 m in 2:00 3 km warm-up 3 km cool-down | **8 km** steady run 6:00 pace | **8 km** form run 5:30–5:45 pace | off |
| **Week 10** | **13 km** steady run 6:20–6:30 pace | off | **8 km** steady run 5:40 pace | **6 speed int.** 400 m in 2:00 3 km warm-up 3 km cool-down | **8 km** steady run 6:00 pace | **8 km** form run 5:30–5:45 pace | off |
| **Week 11** | **16 km** steady run 6:20–6:30 pace | off | **8 km** steady run 5:40 pace | **8 speed int.** 400 m in 2:00 3 km warm-up 3 km cool-down | **13 km** steady run 6:00 pace | **8 km** steady run 5:30–5:45 pace | off |
| **Week 12** | **16 km** steady run 6:20–6:30 pace | off | **6 km** race pace (5:30 pace) | **6 km** race pace (5:30 pace) | **3 km** steady run 6:00 pace | off | **3 km** easy run |
| **FINALE !** | **10 km** RACE DAY! 5:30 pace | | | | | | |

weekly total    long run

| | 60 | | | | | | | | | | | | 60 |
|---|---|---|---|---|---|---|---|---|---|---|---|---|---|
| | 50 | | | | | | | | | | | | 50 |
| | 40 | | | | | | | | | | | | 40 |
| | 30 | | | | | | | | | | | | 30 |
| | 20 | | | | | | | | | | | | 20 |
| | 10 | | | | | | | | | | | | 10 |
| | 0 | | | | | | | | | | | | 0 |
| | wk 1 | wk 2 | wk 3 | wk 4 | wk 5 | wk 6 | wk 7 | wk 8 | wk 9 | wk 10 | wk 11 | wk 12 | |

# 55 minute 10-K
## training program

*miles*

| | SUN | MON | TUES | WED | THURS | FRI | SAT |
|---|---|---|---|---|---|---|---|
| **Week 1** | off | off | 4 miles<br>steady run<br>9:10 pace | 4 hills<br>85% effort<br>2 mi warm-up<br>2 mi cool-down | 4 miles<br>steady run<br>9:50 pace | 3 miles<br>steady run<br>8:55–9:10 pace | off |
| **Week 2** | 4 miles<br>steady run<br>10:00–10:20 pace | off | 4 miles<br>steady run<br>9:10 pace | 5 hills<br>85% effort<br>2 mi warm-up<br>2 mi cool-down | 4 miles<br>steady run<br>9:50 pace | 3 miles<br>steady run<br>8:55–9:10 pace | off |
| **Week 3** | 6 miles<br>steady run<br>10:00–10:20 pace | off | 4 miles<br>steady run<br>9:10 pace | 6 hills<br>85% effort<br>2 mi warm-up<br>2 mi cool-down | 4 miles<br>steady run<br>9:50 pace | 4 miles<br>steady run<br>8:55–9:10 pace | off |
| **Week 4** | 6 miles<br>steady run<br>10:00–10:20 pace | off | 4 miles<br>steady run<br>9:10 pace | 7 hills<br>85% effort<br>2 mi warm-up<br>2 mi cool-down | 4 miles<br>steady run<br>9:50 pace | 4 miles<br>steady run<br>8:55–9:10 pace | off |
| **Week 5** | 8 miles<br>steady run<br>10:00–10:20 pace | off | 5 miles<br>steady run<br>9:10 pace | 8 hills<br>85% effort<br>2 mi warm-up<br>2 mi cool-down | 5 miles<br>steady run<br>9:50 pace | 5 miles<br>steady run<br>8:55–9:10 pace | off |
| **Week 6** | 10 miles<br>steady run<br>10:00–10:20 pace | off | 5 miles<br>steady run<br>9:10 pace | 9 hills<br>85% effort<br>2 mi warm-up<br>2 mi cool-down | 5 miles<br>steady run<br>9:50 pace | 5 miles<br>steady run<br>8:55–9:10 pace | off |
| **Week 7** | 8 miles<br>steady run<br>10:00–10:20 pace | off | 5 miles<br>steady run<br>9:10 pace | 10 hills<br>85% effort<br>2 mi warm-up<br>2 mi cool-down | 4 miles<br>steady run<br>9:50 pace | 4 miles<br>form run<br>8:55–9:10 pace | off |
| **Week 8** | 10 miles<br>steady run<br>10:00–10:20 pace | off | 5 miles<br>steady run<br>9:10 pace | 4 speed int.<br>400 m in 2:00<br>2 mi warm-up<br>2 mi cool-down | 5 miles<br>steady run<br>9:50 pace | 5 miles<br>form run<br>8:55–9:10 pace | off |
| **Week 9** | 10 miles<br>steady run<br>10:00–10:20 pace | off | 5 miles<br>steady run<br>9:10 pace | 5 speed int.<br>400 m in 2:00<br>2 mi warm-up<br>2 mi cool-down | 5 miles<br>steady run<br>9:50 pace | 5 miles<br>form run<br>8:55–9:10 pace | off |
| **Week 10** | 8 miles<br>steady run<br>10:00–10:20 pace | off | 5 miles<br>steady run<br>9:10 pace | 6 speed int.<br>400 m in 2:00<br>2 mi warm-up<br>2 mi cool-down | 5 miles<br>steady run<br>9:50 pace | 5 miles<br>form run<br>8:55–9:10 pace | off |
| **Week 11** | 10 miles<br>steady run<br>10:00–10:20 pace | off | 5 miles<br>steady run<br>9:10 pace | 8 speed int.<br>400 m in 2:00<br>2 mi warm-up<br>2 mi cool-down | 8 miles<br>steady run<br>9:50 pace | 5 miles<br>steady run<br>8:55–9:10 pace | off |
| **Week 12** | 10 miles<br>steady run<br>10:00–10:20 pace | off | 4 miles<br>race pace<br>(8:51 pace) | 4 miles<br>race pace<br>(8:51 pace) | 2 miles<br>steady run<br>9:50 pace | off | 2 miles<br>easy run |
| **FINALE !** | 6.2 miles<br>RACE DAY!<br>8:51 pace | | | | | | |

weekly total   long run

| | wk 1 | wk 2 | wk 3 | wk 4 | wk 5 | wk 6 | wk 7 | wk 8 | wk 9 | wk 10 | wk 11 | wk 12 |
|---|---|---|---|---|---|---|---|---|---|---|---|---|

# 50 minute 10-K
## training program

### *kilometres*

| | SUN | MON | TUES | WED | THURS | FRI | SAT |
|---|---|---|---|---|---|---|---|
| **Week 1** | off | off | 6 km<br>steady run<br>5:10 pace | 4 hills<br>85% effort<br>3 km warm-up<br>3 km cool-down | 6 km<br>steady run<br>5:35 pace | 5 km<br>form/tempo<br>5:00–5:20 pace | off |
| **Week 2** | 6 km<br>steady run<br>5:35–6:00 pace | off | 6 km<br>steady run<br>5:10 pace | 5 hills<br>85% effort<br>3 km warm-up<br>3 km cool-down | 6 km<br>steady run<br>5:35 pace | 5 km<br>form/tempo<br>5:00–5:20 pace | off |
| **Week 3** | 10 km<br>steady run<br>5:35–6:00 pace | off | 6 km<br>steady run<br>5:10 pace | 6 hills<br>85% effort<br>3 km warm-up<br>3 km cool-down | 6 km<br>steady run<br>5:35 pace | 6 km<br>form/tempo<br>5:00–5:20 pace | off |
| **Week 4** | 10 km<br>steady run<br>5:35–6:00 pace | off | 6 km<br>steady run<br>5:10 pace | 7 hills<br>85% effort<br>3 km warm-up<br>3 km cool-down | 6 km<br>steady run<br>5:35 pace | 6 km<br>form/tempo<br>5:00–5:20 pace | off |
| **Week 5** | 13 km<br>steady run<br>5:35–6:00 pace | off | 8 km<br>steady run<br>5:10 pace | 8 hills<br>85% effort<br>3 km warm-up<br>3 km cool-down | 8 km<br>steady run<br>5:35 pace | 8 km<br>form/tempo<br>5:00–5:20 pace | off |
| **Week 6** | 16 km<br>steady run<br>5:35–6:00 pace | off | 8 km<br>steady run<br>5:10 pace | 9 hills<br>85% effort<br>3 km warm-up<br>3 km cool-down | 8 km<br>steady run<br>5:35 pace | 8 km<br>form/tempo<br>5:00–5:20 pace | off |
| **Week 7** | 13 km<br>steady run<br>5:35–6:00 pace | off | 8 km<br>steady run<br>5:10 pace | 10 hills<br>85% effort<br>3 km warm-up<br>3 km cool-down | 6 km<br>steady run<br>5:35 pace | 6 km<br>form/tempo<br>5:00–5:20 pace | off |
| **Week 8** | 16 km<br>steady run<br>5:35–6:00 pace | off | 8 km<br>steady run<br>5:10 pace | 4 speed int.<br>400 m in 1:55<br>3 km warm-up<br>3 km cool-down | 8 km<br>steady run<br>5:35 pace | 8 km<br>form/tempo<br>5:00–5:20 pace | off |
| **Week 9** | 16 km<br>steady run<br>5:35–6:00 pace | off | 8 km<br>steady run<br>5:10 pace | 5 speed int.<br>400 m in 1:55<br>3 km warm-up<br>3 km cool-down | 8 km<br>steady run<br>5:35 pace | 8 km<br>form/tempo<br>5:00–5:20 pace | off |
| **Week 10** | 13 km<br>steady run<br>5:35–6:00 pace | off | 8 km<br>steady run<br>5:10 pace | 6 speed int.<br>400 m in 1:55<br>3 km warm-up<br>3 km cool-down | 8 km<br>steady run<br>5:35 pace | 8 km<br>form/tempo<br>5:00–5:20 pace | off |
| **Week 11** | 16 km<br>steady run<br>5:35–6:00 pace | off | 8 km<br>steady run<br>5:10 pace | 8 speed int.<br>400 m in 1:55<br>3 km warm-up<br>3 km cool-down | 13 km<br>steady run<br>5:35 pace | 8 km<br>form/tempo<br>5:00–5:20 pace | off |
| **Week 12** | 16 km<br>steady run<br>5:35–6:00 pace | off | 6 km<br>race pace<br>(5:00 pace) | 6 km<br>race pace<br>(5:00 pace) | 3 km<br>steady run<br>5:35 pace | off | 3 km<br>easy run |
| **FINALE !** | 10 km<br>RACE DAY!<br>5:00 pace | | | | | | |

**weekly total** · **long run**

# 50 minute 10-K
*training program*

| | SUN | MON | TUES | WED | THURS | FRI | SAT |
|---|---|---|---|---|---|---|---|
| **Week 1** | off | off | 4 miles<br>steady run<br>8:15 pace | 4 hills<br>85% effort<br>2 mi warm-up<br>2 mi cool-down | 4 miles<br>steady run<br>9:00 pace | 3 miles<br>form/tempo<br>8:05–8:35 pace | off |
| **Week 2** | 4 miles<br>steady run<br>9:00–9:30 pace | off | 4 miles<br>steady run<br>8:15 pace | 5 hills<br>85% effort<br>2 mi warm-up<br>2 mi cool-down | 4 miles<br>steady run<br>9:00 pace | 3 miles<br>form/tempo<br>8:05–8:35 pace | off |
| **Week 3** | 6 miles<br>steady run<br>9:00–9:30 pace | off | 4 miles<br>steady run<br>8:15 pace | 6 hills<br>85% effort<br>2 mi warm-up<br>2 mi cool-down | 4 miles<br>steady run<br>9:00 pace | 4 miles<br>form/tempo<br>8:05–8:35 pace | off |
| **Week 4** | 6 miles<br>steady run<br>9:00–9:30 pace | off | 4 miles<br>steady run<br>8:15 pace | 7 hills<br>85% effort<br>2 mi warm-up<br>2 mi cool-down | 4 miles<br>steady run<br>9:00 pace | 4 miles<br>form/tempo<br>8:05–8:35 pace | off |
| **Week 5** | 8 miles<br>steady run<br>9:00–9:30 pace | off | 5 miles<br>steady run<br>8:15 pace | 8 hills<br>85% effort<br>2 mi warm-up<br>2 mi cool-down | 5 miles<br>steady run<br>9:00 pace | 5 miles<br>form/tempo<br>8:05–8:35 pace | off |
| **Week 6** | 10 miles<br>steady run<br>9:00–9:30 pace | off | 5 miles<br>steady run<br>8:15 pace | 9 hills<br>85% effort<br>2 mi warm-up<br>2 mi cool-down | 5 miles<br>steady run<br>9:00 pace | 5 miles<br>form/tempo<br>8:05–8:35 pace | off |
| **Week 7** | 8 miles<br>steady run<br>9:00–9:30 pace | off | 5 miles<br>steady run<br>8:15 pace | 10 hills<br>85% effort<br>2 mi warm-up<br>2 mi cool-down | 4 miles<br>steady run<br>9:00 pace | 4 miles<br>form/tempo<br>8:05–8:35 pace | off |
| **Week 8** | 10 miles<br>steady run<br>9:00–9:30 pace | off | 5 miles<br>steady run<br>8:15 pace | 4 speed int.<br>400 m in 1:55<br>2 mi warm-up<br>2 mi cool-down | 5 miles<br>steady run<br>9:00 pace | 5 miles<br>form/tempo<br>8:05–8:35 pace | off |
| **Week 9** | 10 miles<br>steady run<br>9:00–9:30 pace | off | 5 miles<br>steady run<br>8:15 pace | 5 speed int.<br>400 m in 1:55<br>2 mi warm-up<br>2 mi cool-down | 5 miles<br>steady run<br>9:00 pace | 5 miles<br>form/tempo<br>8:05–8:35 pace | off |
| **Week 10** | 8 miles<br>steady run<br>9:00–9:30 pace | off | 5 miles<br>steady run<br>8:15 pace | 6 speed int.<br>400 m in 1:55<br>2 mi warm-up<br>2 mi cool-down | 5 miles<br>steady run<br>9:00 pace | 5 miles<br>form/tempo<br>8:05–8:35 pace | off |
| **Week 11** | 10 miles<br>steady run<br>9:00–9:30 pace | off | 5 miles<br>steady run<br>8:15 pace | 8 speed int.<br>400 m in 1:55<br>2 mi warm-up<br>2 mi cool-down | 8 miles<br>steady run<br>9:00 pace | 5 miles<br>form/tempo<br>8:05–8:35 pace | off |
| **Week 12** | 10 miles<br>steady run<br>9:00–9:30 pace | off | 4 miles<br>race pace<br>(8:03 pace) | 4 miles<br>race pace<br>(8:03 pace) | 2 miles<br>steady run<br>9:00 pace | off | 2 miles<br>easy run |
| **FINALE !** | 6.2 miles<br>RACE DAY!<br>8:03 pace | | | | | | |

☐ weekly total   ☐ long run

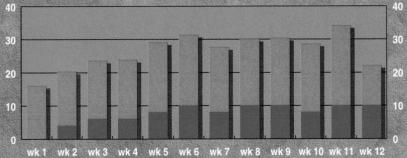

# 48 minute 10-K
## training program

*kilometres*

| | SUN | MON | TUES | WED | THURS | FRI | SAT |
|---|---|---|---|---|---|---|---|
| **Week 1** | off | off | 6 km steady run 5:00 pace | 6 hills 85% effort 3 km warm-up 3 km cool-down | 6 km steady run 5:30 pace | 5 km form/tempo 4:50–5:10 pace | 5 km steady run 5:30 pace |
| **Week 2** | 6 km steady run 5:25–5:45 pace | off | 6 km steady run 5:00 pace | 7 hills 85% effort 3 km warm-up 3 km cool-down | 6 km steady run 5:30 pace | 5 km form/tempo 4:50–5:10 pace | 5 km steady run 5:30 pace |
| **Week 3** | 10 km steady run 5:25–5:45 pace | off | 6 km steady run 5:00 pace | 8 hills 85% effort 3 km warm-up 3 km cool-down | 6 km steady run 5:30 pace | 6 km form/tempo 4:50–5:10 pace | 5 km steady run 5:30 pace |
| **Week 4** | 10 km steady run 5:25–5:45 pace | off | 6 km steady run 5:00 pace | 9 hills 85% effort 3 km warm-up 3 km cool-down | 6 km steady run 5:30 pace | 6 km form/tempo 4:50–5:10 pace | 5 km steady run 5:30 pace |
| **Week 5** | 13 km steady run 5:25–5:45 pace | off | 8 km steady run 5:00 pace | 10 hills 85% effort 3 km warm-up 3 km cool-down | 8 km steady run 5:30 pace | 8 km form/tempo 4:50–5:10 pace | off |
| **Week 6** | 16 km steady run 5:25–5:45 pace | off | 8 km steady run 5:00 pace | 11 hills 85% effort 3 km warm-up 3 km cool-down | 8 km steady run 5:30 pace | 8 km form/tempo 4:50–5:10 pace | 5 km steady run 5:30 pace |
| **Week 7** | 13 km steady run 5:25–5:45 pace | off | 6 km steady run 5:00 pace | 12 hills 85% effort 3 km warm-up 3 km cool-down | 8 km steady run 5:30 pace | 6 km form/tempo 4:50–5:10 pace | off |
| **Week 8** | 16 km steady run 5:25–5:45 pace | off | 8 km steady run 5:00 pace | 4 speed int. 400 m in 1:50 3 km warm-up 3 km cool-down | 8 km steady run 5:30 pace | 8 km form/tempo 4:50–5:10 pace | 5 km steady run 5:30 pace |
| **Week 9** | 19 km steady run 5:25–5:45 pace | off | 8 km steady run 5:00 pace | 5 speed int. 400 m in 1:50 3 km warm-up 3 km cool-down | 8 km steady run 5:30 pace | 8 km form/tempo 4:50–5:10 pace | 5 km steady run 5:30 pace |
| **Week 10** | 22 km steady run 5:25–5:45 pace | off | 8 km steady run 5:00 pace | 6 speed int. 400 m in 1:50 3 km warm-up 3 km cool-down | 8 km steady run 5:30 pace | 8 km form/tempo 4:50–5:10 pace | 5 km steady run 5:30 pace |
| **Week 11** | 26 km steady run 5:25–5:45 pace | off | 8 km steady run 5:00 pace | 8 speed int. 400 m in 1:50 3 km warm-up 3 km cool-down | 8 km steady run 5:30 pace | 8 km form/tempo 4:50–5:10 pace | 6 km steady run 5:30 pace |
| **Week 12** | 13 km steady run 5:25–5:45 pace | off | 8 km race pace (4:48 pace) | 6 km race pace (4:48 pace) | 3 km steady run 5:30 pace | off | 3 km steady run 5:30 pace |
| **FINALE !** | 10 km RACE DAY! 4:48 pace | | | | | | |

weekly total    long run

# *miles*

# 48 minute 10-K
## *training program*

| | SUN | MON | TUES | WED | THURS | FRI | SAT |
|---|---|---|---|---|---|---|---|
| **Week 1** | off | off | 4 miles<br>steady run<br>8:05 pace | 6 hills<br>85% effort<br>2 mi warm-up<br>2 mi cool-down | 4 miles<br>steady run<br>8:45 pace | 3 miles<br>form/tempo<br>7:45–8:15 pace | 3 miles<br>steady run<br>8:45 pace |
| **Week 2** | 4 miles<br>steady run<br>8:45–9:15 pace | off | 4 miles<br>steady run<br>8:05 pace | 7 hills<br>85% effort<br>2 mi warm-up<br>2 mi cool-down | 4 miles<br>steady run<br>8:45 pace | 3 miles<br>form/tempo<br>7:45–8:15 pace | 3 miles<br>steady run<br>8:45 pace |
| **Week 3** | 6 miles<br>steady run<br>8:45–9:15 pace | off | 4 miles<br>steady run<br>8:05 pace | 8 hills<br>85% effort<br>2 mi warm-up<br>2 mi cool-down | 4 miles<br>steady run<br>8:45 pace | 4 miles<br>form/tempo<br>7:45–8:15 pace | 3 miles<br>steady run<br>8:45 pace |
| **Week 4** | 6 miles<br>steady run<br>8:45–9:15 pace | off | 4 miles<br>steady run<br>8:05 pace | 9 hills<br>85% effort<br>2 mi warm-up<br>2 mi cool-down | 4 miles<br>steady run<br>8:45 pace | 4 miles<br>form/tempo<br>7:45–8:15 pace | 3 miles<br>steady run<br>8:45 pace |
| **Week 5** | 8 miles<br>steady run<br>8:45–9:15 pace | off | 5 miles<br>steady run<br>8:05 pace | 10 hills<br>85% effort<br>2 mi warm-up<br>2 mi cool-down | 5 miles<br>steady run<br>8:45 pace | 5 miles<br>form/tempo<br>7:45–8:15 pace | off |
| **Week 6** | 10 miles<br>steady run<br>8:45–9:15 pace | off | 5 miles<br>steady run<br>8:05 pace | 11 hills<br>85% effort<br>2 mi warm-up<br>2 mi cool-down | 5 miles<br>steady run<br>8:45 pace | 5 miles<br>form/tempo<br>7:45–8:15 pace | 3 miles<br>steady run<br>8:45 pace |
| **Week 7** | 8 miles<br>steady run<br>8:45–9:15 pace | off | 4 miles<br>steady run<br>8:05 pace | 12 hills<br>85% effort<br>2 mi warm-up<br>2 mi cool-down | 5 miles<br>steady run<br>8:45 pace | 4 miles<br>form/tempo<br>7:45–8:15 pace | off |
| **Week 8** | 10 miles<br>steady run<br>8:45–9:15 pace | off | 5 miles<br>steady run<br>8:05 pace | 4 speed int.<br>400 m in 1:50<br>2 mi warm-up<br>2 mi cool-down | 5 miles<br>steady run<br>8:45 pace | 5 miles<br>form/tempo<br>7:45–8:15 pace | 3 miles<br>steady run<br>8:45 pace |
| **Week 9** | 12 miles<br>steady run<br>8:45–9:15 pace | off | 5 miles<br>steady run<br>8:05 pace | 5 speed int.<br>400 m in 1:50<br>2 mi warm-up<br>2 mi cool-down | 5 miles<br>steady run<br>8:45 pace | 5 miles<br>form/tempo<br>7:45–8:15 pace | 3 miles<br>steady run<br>8:45 pace |
| **Week 10** | 14 miles<br>steady run<br>8:45–9:15 pace | off | 5 miles<br>steady run<br>8:05 pace | 6 speed int.<br>400 m in 1:50<br>2 mi warm-up<br>2 mi cool-down | 5 miles<br>steady run<br>8:45 pace | 5 miles<br>form/tempo<br>7:45–8:15 pace | 3 miles<br>steady run<br>8:45 pace |
| **Week 11** | 16 miles<br>steady run<br>8:45–9:15 pace | off | 5 miles<br>steady run<br>8:05 pace | 8 speed int.<br>400 m in 1:50<br>2 mi warm-up<br>2 mi cool-down | 5 miles<br>steady run<br>8:45 pace | 5 miles<br>form/tempo<br>7:45–8:15 pace | 4 miles<br>steady run<br>8:45 pace |
| **Week 12** | 8 miles<br>steady run<br>8:45–9:15 pace | off | 5 miles<br>race pace<br>(7:43 pace) | 4 miles<br>race pace<br>(7:43 pace) | 2 miles<br>steady run<br>8:45 pace | off | 2 miles<br>steady run<br>8:45 pace |
| **FINALE !** | 6.2 miles<br>RACE DAY!<br>7:43 pace | | | | | | |

▢ **weekly total**  ▮ **long run**

Bar chart — weekly total and long run mileage for wk 1 through wk 12, scale 0–50.

**179**

# 44 minute 10-K
## training program

| | SUN | MON | TUES | WED | THURS | FRI | SAT |
|---|---|---|---|---|---|---|---|
| **Week 1** | off | off | 6 km<br>steady run<br>4:10 pace | 4 hills<br>85% effort<br>3 km warm-up<br>3 km cool-down | 5 km<br>steady run<br>4:55 pace | 6 km<br>tempo run<br>4:25–4:45 pace | 5 km<br>steady run<br>5:00 pace |
| **Week 2** | 10 km<br>steady run<br>5:00–5:15 pace | off | 6 km<br>steady run<br>4:30 pace | 5 hills<br>85% effort<br>3 km warm-up<br>3 km cool-down | 5 km<br>steady run<br>5:00 pace | 6 km<br>tempo run<br>4:25–4:45 pace | 5 km<br>steady run<br>5:00 pace |
| **Week 3** | 10 km<br>steady run<br>5:00–5:15 pace | off | 6 km<br>steady run<br>4:30 pace | 6 hills<br>85% effort<br>3 km warm-up<br>3 km cool-down | 6 km<br>steady run<br>5:00 pace | 5 km<br>tempo run<br>4:25–4:45 pace | 6 km<br>steady run<br>5:00 pace |
| **Week 4** | 13 km<br>steady run<br>5:00–5:15 pace | off | 6 km<br>steady run<br>4:30 pace | 7 hills<br>85% effort<br>3 km warm-up<br>3 km cool-down | 5 km<br>steady run<br>5:00 pace | 6 km<br>tempo run<br>4:25–4:45 pace | 6 km<br>steady run<br>5:00 pace |
| **Week 5** | 16 km<br>steady run<br>5:00–5:15 pace | off | 8 km<br>steady run<br>4:30 pace | 8 hills<br>85% effort<br>3 km warm-up<br>3 km cool-down | 8 km<br>steady run<br>5:00 pace | 8 km<br>tempo run<br>4:25–4:45 pace | off |
| **Week 6** | 16 km<br>steady run<br>5:00–5:15 pace | off | 8 km<br>steady run<br>4:30 pace | 9 hills<br>85% effort<br>3 km warm-up<br>3 km cool-down | 8 km<br>steady run<br>5:00 pace | 8 km<br>tempo run<br>4:25–4:45 pace | 5 km<br>steady run<br>5:00 pace |
| **Week 7** | 19 km<br>steady run<br>5:00–5:15 pace | off | 8 km<br>steady run<br>4:30 pace | 10 hills<br>85% effort<br>3 km warm-up<br>3 km cool-down | 6 km<br>steady run<br>5:00 pace | 6 km<br>tempo run<br>4:25–4:45 pace | off |
| **Week 8** | 16 km<br>steady run<br>5:00–5:15 pace | off | 8 km<br>steady run<br>4:30 pace | 4 speed int.<br>400 m in 1:40<br>3 km warm-up<br>3 km cool-down | 8 km<br>steady run<br>5:00 pace | 8 km<br>tempo run<br>4:25–4:45 pace | 5 km<br>steady run<br>5:00 pace |
| **Week 9** | 19 km<br>steady run<br>5:00–5:15 pace | off | 8 km<br>steady run<br>4:30 pace | 5 speed int.<br>400 m in 1:40<br>3 km warm-up<br>3 km cool-down | 8 km<br>steady run<br>5:00 pace | 8 km<br>tempo run<br>4:25–4:45 pace | 5 km<br>steady run<br>5:00 pace |
| **Week 10** | 22 km<br>steady run<br>5:00–5:15 pace | off | 8 km<br>steady run<br>4:30 pace | 6 speed int.<br>400 m in 1:40<br>3 km warm-up<br>3 km cool-down | 6 km<br>steady run<br>5:00 pace | 8 km<br>tempo run<br>4:25–4:45 pace | 5 km<br>steady run<br>5:00 pace |
| **Week 11** | 26 km<br>steady run<br>5:00–5:15 pace | off | 13 km<br>steady run<br>4:30 pace | 8 speed int.<br>400 m in 1:40<br>3 km warm-up<br>3 km cool-down | 8 km<br>steady run<br>5:00 pace | 8 km<br>tempo run<br>4:25–4:45 pace | 6 km<br>steady run<br>5:00 pace |
| **Week 12** | 13 km<br>steady run<br>5:00–5:15 pace | off | 6 km<br>race pace<br>(4:24 pace) | 6 km<br>race pace<br>(4:24 pace) | 3 km<br>steady run<br>5:00 pace | off | 3 km<br>steady run<br>5:00 pace |
| **FINALE!** | | 10 km<br>RACE DAY!<br>4:24 pace | | | | | |

weekly total        long run

| | 80 | 70 | 60 | 50 | 40 | 30 | 20 | 10 | 0 |
|---|---|---|---|---|---|---|---|---|---|

wk 1   wk 2   wk 3   wk 4   wk 5   wk 6   wk 7   wk 8   wk 9   wk 10   wk 11   wk 12

# miles

# 44 minute 10-K
## training program

| | SUN | MON | TUES | WED | THURS | FRI | SAT |
|---|---|---|---|---|---|---|---|
| **Week 1** | off | off | 4 miles<br>steady run<br>7:15 pace | 4 hills<br>85% effort<br>2 mi warm-up<br>2 mi cool-down | 3 miles<br>steady run<br>8:00 pace | 4 miles<br>tempo run<br>7:10–7:40 pace | 3 miles<br>steady run<br>8:00 pace |
| **Week 2** | 6 miles<br>steady run<br>8:00–8:30 pace | off | 4 miles<br>steady run<br>7:15 pace | 5 hills<br>85% effort<br>2 mi warm-up<br>2 mi cool-down | 3 miles<br>steady run<br>8:00 pace | 4 miles<br>tempo run<br>7:10–7:40 pace | 3 miles<br>steady run<br>8:00 pace |
| **Week 3** | 6 miles<br>steady run<br>8:00–8:30 pace | off | 4 miles<br>steady run<br>7:15 pace | 6 hills<br>85% effort<br>2 mi warm-up<br>2 mi cool-down | 4 miles<br>steady run<br>8:00 pace | 3 miles<br>tempo run<br>7:10–7:40 pace | 4 miles<br>steady run<br>8:00 pace |
| **Week 4** | 8 miles<br>steady run<br>8:00–8:30 pace | off | 4 miles<br>steady run<br>7:15 pace | 7 hills<br>85% effort<br>2 mi warm-up<br>2 mi cool-down | 3 miles<br>steady run<br>8:00 pace | 4 miles<br>tempo run<br>7:10–7:40 pace | 4 miles<br>steady run<br>8:00 pace |
| **Week 5** | 10 miles<br>steady run<br>8:00–8:30 pace | off | 5 miles<br>steady run<br>7:15 pace | 8 hills<br>85% effort<br>2 mi warm-up<br>2 mi cool-down | 5 miles<br>steady run<br>8:00 pace | 5 miles<br>tempo run<br>7:10–7:40 pace | off |
| **Week 6** | 10 miles<br>steady run<br>8:00–8:30 pace | off | 5 miles<br>steady run<br>7:15 pace | 9 hills<br>85% effort<br>2 mi warm-up<br>2 mi cool-down | 5 miles<br>steady run<br>8:00 pace | 5 miles<br>tempo run<br>7:10–7:40 pace | 3 miles<br>steady run<br>8:00 pace |
| **Week 7** | 12 miles<br>steady run<br>8:00–8:30 pace | off | 5 miles<br>steady run<br>7:15 pace | 10 hills<br>85% effort<br>2 mi warm-up<br>2 mi cool-down | 4 miles<br>steady run<br>8:00 pace | 4 miles<br>tempo run<br>7:10–7:40 pace | off |
| **Week 8** | 10 miles<br>steady run<br>8:00–8:30 pace | off | 5 miles<br>steady run<br>7:15 pace | 4 speed int.<br>400 m in 1:40<br>2 mi warm-up<br>2 mi cool-down | 5 miles<br>steady run<br>8:00 pace | 5 miles<br>tempo run<br>7:10–7:40 pace | 3 miles<br>steady run<br>8:00 pace |
| **Week 9** | 12 miles<br>steady run<br>8:00–8:30 pace | off | 5 miles<br>steady run<br>7:15 pace | 5 speed int.<br>400 m in 1:40<br>2 mi warm-up<br>2 mi cool-down | 5 miles<br>steady run<br>8:00 pace | 5 miles<br>tempo run<br>7:10–7:40 pace | 3 miles<br>steady run<br>8:00 pace |
| **Week 10** | 14 miles<br>steady run<br>8:00–8:30 pace | off | 5 miles<br>steady run<br>7:15 pace | 6 speed int.<br>400 m in 1:40<br>2 mi warm-up<br>2 mi cool-down | 4 miles<br>steady run<br>8:00 pace | 5 miles<br>tempo run<br>7:10–7:40 pace | 3 miles<br>steady run<br>8:00 pace |
| **Week 11** | 16 miles<br>steady run<br>8:00–8:30 pace | off | 8 miles<br>steady run<br>7:15 pace | 8 speed int.<br>400 m in 1:40<br>2 mi warm-up<br>2 mi cool-down | 5 miles<br>steady run<br>8:00 pace | 5 miles<br>tempo run<br>7:10–7:40 pace | 4 miles<br>steady run<br>8:00 pace |
| **Week 12** | 8 miles<br>steady run<br>8:00–8:30 pace | off | 4 miles<br>race pace<br>(7:05 pace) | 4 miles<br>race pace<br>(7:05 pace) | 2 miles<br>steady run<br>8:00 pace | off | 2 miles<br>steady run<br>8:00 pace |
| **FINALE !** | 6.2 miles<br>RACE DAY!<br>7:05 pace | | | | | | |

weekly total     long run

181

# 40 minute 10-K
*training program*

### kilometres

| | SUN | MON | TUES | WED | THURS | FRI | SAT |
|---|---|---|---|---|---|---|---|
| **Week 1** | off | off | 6 km<br>steady run<br>4:10 pace | 5 hills<br>85% effort<br>3 km warm-up<br>3 km cool-down | 8 km<br>steady run<br>4:55 pace | 8 km<br>form/tempo<br>4:00–4:20 pace | 8 km<br>steady run<br>4:55 pace |
| **Week 2** | 10 km<br>steady run<br>4:40–5:00 pace | off | 6 km<br>steady run<br>4:10 pace | 6 hills<br>85% effort<br>3 km warm-up<br>3 km cool-down | 8 km<br>steady run<br>4:55 pace | 8 km<br>form/tempo<br>4:00–4:20 pace | 8 km<br>steady run<br>4:55 pace |
| **Week 3** | 13 km<br>steady run<br>4:40–5:00 pace | off | 6 km<br>steady run<br>4:10 pace | 7 hills<br>85% effort<br>3 km warm-up<br>3 km cool-down | 13 km<br>steady run<br>4:55 pace | 13 km<br>form/tempo<br>4:00–4:20 pace | 6 km<br>steady run<br>4:55 pace |
| **Week 4** | 16 km<br>steady run<br>4:40–5:00 pace | off | 6 km<br>steady run<br>4:10 pace | 8 hills<br>85% effort<br>3 km warm-up<br>3 km cool-down | 8 km<br>steady run<br>4:55 pace | 13 km<br>form/tempo<br>4:00–4:20 pace | 8 km<br>steady run<br>4:55 pace |
| **Week 5** | 19 km<br>steady run<br>4:40–5:00 pace | off | 8 km<br>steady run<br>4:10 pace | 9 hills<br>85% effort<br>3 km warm-up<br>3 km cool-down | 13 km<br>steady run<br>4:55 pace | 13 km<br>form/tempo<br>4:00–4:20 pace | 8 km<br>steady run<br>4:55 pace |
| **Week 6** | 22 km<br>steady run<br>4:40–5:00 pace | off | 10 km<br>steady run<br>4:10 pace | 10 hills<br>85% effort<br>3 km warm-up<br>3 km cool-down | 16 km<br>steady run<br>4:55 pace | 13 km<br>form/tempo<br>4:00–4:20 pace | 8 km<br>steady run<br>4:55 pace |
| **Week 7** | 26 km<br>steady run<br>4:40–5:00 pace | off | 8 km<br>steady run<br>4:10 pace | 4 speed int.<br>400 m in 90 sec.<br>3 km warm-up<br>3 km cool-down | 16 km<br>steady run<br>4:55 pace | 13 km<br>form/tempo<br>4:00–4:20 pace | 8 km<br>steady run<br>4:55 pace |
| **Week 8** | 19 km<br>steady run<br>4:40–5:00 pace | off | 8 km<br>steady run<br>4:10 pace | 5 speed int.<br>400 m in 90 sec.<br>3 km warm-up<br>3 km cool-down | 16 km<br>steady run<br>4:55 pace | 13 km<br>form/tempo<br>4:00–4:20 pace | 8 km<br>steady run<br>4:55 pace |
| **Week 9** | 26 km<br>steady run<br>4:40–5:00 pace | off | 8 km<br>steady run<br>4:10 pace | 6 speed int.<br>400 m in 90 sec.<br>3 km warm-up<br>3 km cool-down | 16 km<br>steady run<br>4:55 pace | 10 km<br>form/tempo<br>4:00–4:20 pace | off |
| **Week 10** | 26 km<br>steady run<br>4:40–5:00 pace | off | 8 km<br>steady run<br>4:10 pace | 5 speed int.<br>800 m in 3:00<br>3 km warm-up<br>3 km cool-down | 16 km<br>steady run<br>4:55 pace | 8 km<br>form/tempo<br>4:00–4:20 pace | 8 km<br>steady run<br>4:55 pace |
| **Week 11** | 26 km<br>steady run<br>4:40–5:00 pace | off | 8 km<br>steady run<br>4:10 pace | 6 speed int.<br>800 m in 3:00<br>3 km warm-up<br>3 km cool-down | 8 km<br>steady run<br>4:55 pace | off | off |
| **Week 12** | 16 km<br>steady run<br>4:40–5:00 pace | off | 6 km<br>race pace<br>(4:00 pace) | 6 km<br>race pace<br>(4:00 pace) | 6 km<br>steady run<br>5:00 pace | off | 3 km<br>steady run<br>4:55 pace |
| **FINALE !** | 10 km<br>RACE DAY!<br>4:00 pace | | | | | | |

■ weekly total   ■ long run

wk 1  wk 2  wk 3  wk 4  wk 5  wk 6  wk 7  wk 8  wk 9  wk 10  wk 11  wk 12

*miles*

# 40 minute 10-K
*training program*

| | SUN | MON | TUES | WED | THURS | FRI | SAT |
|---|---|---|---|---|---|---|---|
| **Week 1** | off | off | 4 miles steady run 6:45 pace | 5 hills 85% effort 2 mi warm-up 2 mi cool-down | 5 miles steady run 7:50 pace | 5 miles form/tempo 6:30–7:00 pace | 5 miles steady run 7:50 pace |
| **Week 2** | 6 miles steady run 7:30–8:00 pace | off | 4 miles steady run 6:45 pace | 6 hills 85% effort 2 mi warm-up 2 mi cool-down | 5 miles steady run 7:50 pace | 5 miles form/tempo 6:30–7:00 pace | 5 miles steady run 7:50 pace |
| **Week 3** | 8 miles steady run 7:30–8:00 pace | off | 4 miles steady run 6:45 pace | 7 hills 85% effort 2 mi warm-up 2 mi cool-down | 8 miles steady run 7:50 pace | 8 miles form/tempo 6:30–7:00 pace | 4 miles steady run 7:50 pace |
| **Week 4** | 10 miles steady run 7:30–8:00 pace | off | 4 miles steady run 6:45 pace | 8 hills 85% effort 2 mi warm-up 2 mi cool-down | 8 miles steady run 7:50 pace | 8 miles form/tempo 6:30–7:00 pace | 5 miles steady run 7:50 pace |
| **Week 5** | 12 miles steady run 7:30–8:00 pace | off | 5 miles steady run 6:45 pace | 9 hills 85% effort 2 mi warm-up 2 mi cool-down | 8 miles steady run 7:50 pace | 8 miles form/tempo 6:30–7:00 pace | 5 miles steady run 7:50 pace |
| **Week 6** | 14 miles steady run 7:30–8:00 pace | off | 6 miles steady run 6:45 pace | 10 hills 85% effort 2 mi warm-up 2 mi cool-down | 8 miles steady run 7:50 pace | 8 miles form/tempo 6:30–7:00 pace | 5 miles steady run 7:50 pace |
| **Week 7** | 16 miles steady run 7:30–8:00 pace | off | 5 miles steady run 6:45 pace | 4 speed int. 400 m in 90 sec. 2 mi warm-up 2 mi cool-down | 10 miles steady run 7:50 pace | 8 miles form/tempo 6:30–7:00 pace | 5 miles steady run 7:50 pace |
| **Week 8** | 12 miles steady run 7:30–8:00 pace | off | 5 miles steady run 6:45 pace | 5 speed int. 400 m in 90 sec. 2 mi warm-up 2 mi cool-down | 10 miles steady run 7:50 pace | 8 miles form/tempo 6:30–7:00 pace | 5 miles steady run 7:50 pace |
| **Week 9** | 16 miles steady run 7:30–8:00 pace | off | 5 miles steady run 6:45 pace | 6 speed int. 400 m in 90 sec. 2 mi warm-up 2 mi cool-down | 10 miles steady run 7:50 pace | 6 miles form/tempo 6:30–7:00 pace | off |
| **Week 10** | 16 miles steady run 7:30–8:00 pace | off | 5 miles steady run 6:45 pace | 5 speed int. 800 m in 3:00 2 mi warm-up 2 mi cool-down | 10 miles steady run 7:50 pace | 5 miles form/tempo 6:30–7:00 pace | 5 miles steady run 7:50 pace |
| **Week 11** | 16 miles steady run 7:30–8:00 pace | off | 5 miles steady run 6:45 pace | 6 speed int. 800 m in 3:00 2 mi warm-up 2 mi cool-down | 5 miles steady run 7:50 pace | off | off |
| **Week 12** | 10 miles steady run 7:30–8:00 pace | off | 4 miles race pace (6:26 pace) | 4 miles race pace (6:26 pace) | 4 miles steady run 8:00 pace | off | 2 miles steady run 7:50 pace |
| **FINALE !** | 6.2 miles RACE DAY! 6:26 pace | | | | | | |

□ weekly total   ■ long run

# 38 minute 10-K
## training program

**kilometres**

| | SUN | MON | TUES | WED | THURS | FRI | SAT |
|---|---|---|---|---|---|---|---|
| **Week 1** | off | off | 6 km steady run 4:00 pace | 5 hills 85% effort 3 km warm-up 3 km cool-down | 8 km steady run 4:45 pace | 8 km form/tempo 3:50–4:05 pace | 8 km steady run 4:45 pace |
| **Week 2** | 10 km steady run 4:30–4:50 pace | off | 6 km steady run 4:00 pace | 6 hills 85% effort 3 km warm-up 3 km cool-down | 8 km steady run 4:45 pace | 8 km form/tempo 3:50–4:05 pace | 8 km steady run 4:45 pace |
| **Week 3** | 13 km steady run 4:30–4:50 pace | off | 6 km steady run 4:00 pace | 7 hills 85% effort 3 km warm-up 3 km cool-down | 13 km steady run 4:45 pace | 13 km form/tempo 3:50–4:05 pace | 6 km steady run 4:45 pace |
| **Week 4** | 16 km steady run 4:30–4:50 pace | off | 6 km steady run 4:00 pace | 8 hills 85% effort 3 km warm-up 3 km cool-down | 13 km steady run 4:45 pace | 13 km form/tempo 3:50–4:05 pace | 8 km steady run 4:45 pace |
| **Week 5** | 19 km steady run 4:30–4:50 pace | off | 8 km steady run 4:00 pace | 9 hills 85% effort 3 km warm-up 3 km cool-down | 13 km steady run 4:45 pace | 13 km form/tempo 3:50–4:05 pace | 8 km steady run 4:45 pace |
| **Week 6** | 22 km steady run 4:30–4:50 pace | off | 10 km steady run 4:00 pace | 10 hills 85% effort 3 km warm-up 3 km cool-down | 16 km steady run 4:45 pace | 16 km form/tempo 3:50–4:05 pace | 6 km steady run 4:45 pace |
| **Week 7** | 24 km steady run 4:30–4:50 pace | off | 10 km steady run 4:00 pace | 4 speed int. 400 m in 85 sec. 3 km warm-up 3 km cool-down | 16 km steady run 4:45 pace | 16 km form/tempo 3:50–4:05 pace | 8 km steady run 4:45 pace |
| **Week 8** | 19 km steady run 4:30–4:50 pace | off | 10 km steady run 4:00 pace | 5 speed int. 400 m in 85 sec. 3 km warm-up 3 km cool-down | 16 km steady run 4:45 pace | 16 km form/tempo 3:50–4:05 pace | 8 km steady run 4:45 pace |
| **Week 9** | 29 km steady run 4:30–4:50 pace | off | 13 km steady run 4:00 pace | 6 speed int. 400 m in 85 sec. 3 km warm-up 3 km cool-down | 13 km steady run 4:45 pace | 16 km form/tempo 3:50–4:05 pace | 8 km steady run 4:45 pace |
| **Week 10** | 29 km steady run 4:30–4:50 pace | off | 13 km steady run 4:00 pace | 5 speed int. 800 m in 2:50 3 km warm-up 3 km cool-down | 13 km steady run 4:45 pace | 16 km form/tempo 3:50–4:05 pace | 8 km steady run 4:45 pace |
| **Week 11** | 29 km steady run 4:30–4:50 pace | off | 8 km steady run 4:00 pace | 6 speed int. 800 m in 2:50 3 km warm-up 3 km cool-down | 8 km steady run 4:45 pace | 13 km form/tempo 3:50–4:05 pace | off |
| **Week 12** | 16 km steady run 4:30–4:50 pace | off | 6 km race pace (3:48 pace) | 6 km race pace (3:48 pace) | 6 km steady run 4:45 pace | off | 3 km steady run 4:45 pace |
| **FINALE !** | | 10 km RACE DAY! 3:48 pace | | | | | |

■ weekly total  ■ long run

# *miles*

# 38 minute 10-K
## *training program*

| | SUN | MON | TUES | WED | THURS | FRI | SAT |
|---|---|---|---|---|---|---|---|
| **Week 1** | off | off | 4 miles<br>steady run<br>6:30 pace | 5 hills<br>85% effort<br>2 mi warm-up<br>2 mi cool-down | 5 miles<br>steady run<br>7:40 pace | 5 miles<br>form/tempo<br>6:10–6:40 pace | 5 miles<br>steady run<br>7:40 pace |
| **Week 2** | 6 miles<br>steady run<br>7:15–7:45 pace | off | 4 miles<br>steady run<br>6:30 pace | 6 hills<br>85% effort<br>2 mi warm-up<br>2 mi cool-down | 5 miles<br>steady run<br>7:40 pace | 5 miles<br>form/tempo<br>6:10–6:40 pace | 5 miles<br>steady run<br>7:40 pace |
| **Week 3** | 8 miles<br>steady run<br>7:15–7:45 pace | off | 4 miles<br>steady run<br>6:30 pace | 7 hills<br>85% effort<br>2 mi warm-up<br>2 mi cool-down | 8 miles<br>steady run<br>7:40 pace | 8 miles<br>form/tempo<br>6:10–6:40 pace | 4 miles<br>steady run<br>7:40 pace |
| **Week 4** | 10 miles<br>steady run<br>7:15–7:45 pace | off | 4 miles<br>steady run<br>6:30 pace | 8 hills<br>85% effort<br>2 mi warm-up<br>2 mi cool-down | 8 miles<br>steady run<br>7:40 pace | 8 miles<br>form/tempo<br>6:10–6:40 pace | 5 miles<br>steady run<br>7:40 pace |
| **Week 5** | 12 miles<br>steady run<br>7:15–7:45 pace | off | 5 miles<br>steady run<br>6:30 pace | 9 hills<br>85% effort<br>2 mi warm-up<br>2 mi cool-down | 8 miles<br>steady run<br>7:40 pace | 8 miles<br>form/tempo<br>6:10–6:40 pace | 5 miles<br>steady run<br>7:40 pace |
| **Week 6** | 14 miles<br>steady run<br>7:15–7:45 pace | off | 6 miles<br>steady run<br>6:30 pace | 10 hills<br>85% effort<br>2 mi warm-up<br>2 mi cool-down | 10 miles<br>steady run<br>7:40 pace | 10 miles<br>form/tempo<br>6:10–6:40 pace | 4 miles<br>steady run<br>7:40 pace |
| **Week 7** | 15 miles<br>steady run<br>7:15–7:45 pace | off | 6 miles<br>steady run<br>6:30 pace | 4 speed int.<br>400 m in 85 sec.<br>2 mi warm-up<br>2 mi cool-down | 10 miles<br>steady run<br>7:40 pace | 10 miles<br>form/tempo<br>6:10–6:40 pace | 5 miles<br>steady run<br>7:40 pace |
| **Week 8** | 12 miles<br>steady run<br>7:15–7:45 pace | off | 6 miles<br>steady run<br>6:30 pace | 5 speed int.<br>400 m in 85 sec.<br>2 mi warm-up<br>2 mi cool-down | 10 miles<br>steady run<br>7:40 pace | 10 miles<br>form/tempo<br>6:10–6:40 pace | 5 miles<br>steady run<br>7:40 pace |
| **Week 9** | 16 miles<br>steady run<br>7:15–7:45 pace | off | 8 miles<br>steady run<br>6:30 pace | 6 speed int.<br>400 m in 85 sec.<br>2 mi warm-up<br>2 mi cool-down | 8 miles<br>steady run<br>7:40 pace | 10 miles<br>form/tempo<br>6:10–6:40 pace | 5 miles<br>steady run<br>7:40 pace |
| **Week 10** | 16 miles<br>steady run<br>7:15–7:45 pace | off | 8 miles<br>steady run<br>6:30 pace | 5 speed int.<br>800 m in 2:50<br>2 mi warm-up<br>2 mi cool-down | 8 miles<br>steady run<br>7:40 pace | 10 miles<br>form/tempo<br>6:10–6:40 pace | 5 miles<br>steady run<br>7:40 pace |
| **Week 11** | 16 miles<br>steady run<br>7:15–7:45 pace | off | 5 miles<br>steady run<br>6:30 pace | 6 speed int.<br>800 m in 2:50<br>2 mi warm-up<br>2 mi cool-down | 5 miles<br>steady run<br>7:40 pace | 8 miles<br>form/tempo<br>6:10–6:40 pace | off |
| **Week 12** | 10 miles<br>steady run<br>7:15–7:45 pace | off | 4 miles<br>race pace<br>(6:07 pace) | 4 miles<br>race pace<br>(6:07 pace) | 4 miles<br>steady run<br>7:40 pace | off | 2 miles<br>steady run<br>7:40 pace |
| **FINALE !** | 6.2 miles<br>RACE DAY!<br>6:07 pace | | | | | | |

☐ **weekly total**   ☐ **long run**

wk 1  wk 2  wk 3  wk 4  wk 5  wk 6  wk 7  wk 8  wk 9  wk 10  wk 11  wk 12

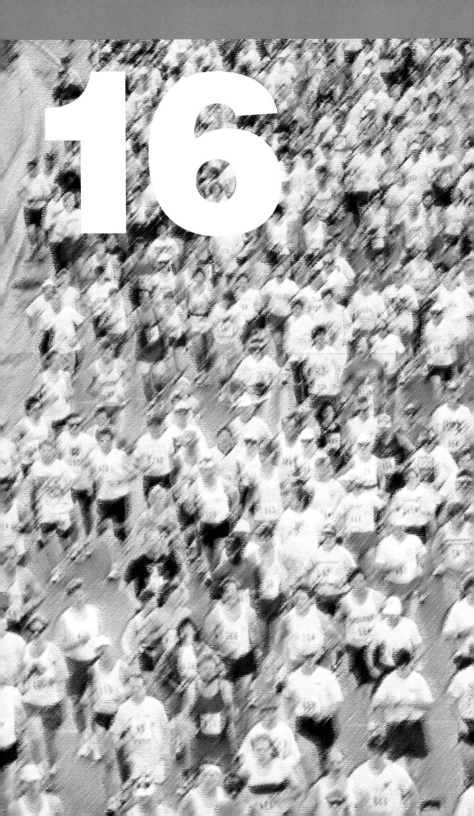

# The Half-Marathon

"I'm only running the half-marathon," is a familiar quote I hear the day before many marathons across the country. Let's set the record straight: the half-marathon is not half a race, and it is not called "only the half-marathon"; it is a challenging distance that gives most folks an equal sense of accomplishment as the full marathon.

Occasionally, I would like to tell runners not to run half-marathons that are attached to full marathons for the very reason that the runners often think they have only run half a race. There are, however, many positive reasons to run them: in most cases, the half-marathon and the marathon start and finish at the same spot, and for running half the distance you get the same goodies at the finish, the same cheering finish-line crowd, the same T-shirt and the same good company to share your celebration.

Some folks really enjoy the half-marathon distance; it challenges them but requires far less training and recovery than the marathon. Training for a half-marathon requires going beyond normal fitness running—it requires some additional time and commitment—but the celebration of the finish line is well worth the effort. The introduction into longer runs gets us back to the basics of long slow runs and the delights that come from doing them. We discover that running can be social, is great for burning fat and awakens us both mentally and physically.

The training schedules on the following pages will help you prepare for a half-marathon. Choose the schedule that best reflects your targeted finish time. There are two schedules for each time goal: the first one presents the training distances in miles; the second in kilometres. A simple bar graph at the bottom of each page summarizes weekly changes in the distance of the long (Sunday) run and in the total weekly distance.

The half marathon is a serious distance—you must take your training seriously—so stick to the program. More is not necessarily better.

# To complete a half-marathon
*training program*     *kilometres*

| | SUN | MON | TUES | WED | THURS | FRI | SAT |
|---|---|---|---|---|---|---|---|
| **Week 1** | **7 km** long, slow run run 10 min/ walk 1 min | off | **4 km** steady run | **3 km** steady run | **3 km** steady run | off | **3 km** steady easy run |
| **Week 2** | **7 km** long, slow run run 10 min/ walk 1 min | off | **4 km** steady run | **3 km** steady run | **4 km** steady run | off | **3 km** steady easy run |
| **Week 3** | **7 km** long, slow run run 10 min/ walk 1 min | off | **3 km** steady run | **4 km** steady run | **3 km** steady run | off | **4 km** steady easy run |
| **Week 4** | **9 km** long, slow run run 10 min/ walk 1 min | off | **4 km** steady run | **4 km** steady run | **3 km** steady run | off | **3 km** steady easy run |
| **Week 5** | **9 km** long, slow run run 10 min/ walk 1 min | off | **5 km** steady run | **3 km** steady run | **4 km** steady run | off | **3 km** steady easy run |
| **Week 6** | **10 km** long, slow run run 10 min/ walk 1 mn | off | **4 km** steady run | **3 hills** 85% effort 3 km warm-up 3 km cool-down | **5 km** steady run | off | **3 km** steady easy run |
| **Week 7** | **10 km** long, slow run run 10 min/ walk 1 min | off | **4 km** steady run | **4 hills** 85% effort 3 km warm-up 3 km cool-down | **5 km** steady run | off | **4 km** steady easy run |
| **Week 8** | **12 km** long, slow run run 10 min/ walk 1 min | off | **4 km** steady run | **5 hills** 85% effort 3 km warm-up 3 km cool-down | **6 km** steady run | off | **4 km** steady easy run |

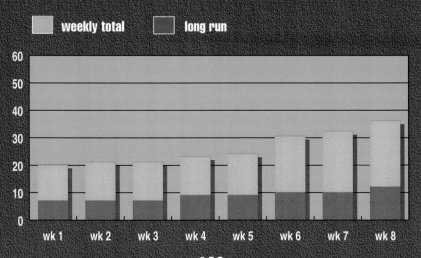

■ weekly total     ■ long run

# kilometres

## To complete a half-marathon
### training program

| | SUN | MON | TUES | WED | THURS | FRI | SAT |
|---|---|---|---|---|---|---|---|
| **Week 9** | **14 km** long, slow run run 10 min/ walk 1 min | off | **4 km** steady run | **6 hills** 85% effort 3 km warm-up 3 km cool-down | **6 km** steady run | off | **5 km** steady easy run |
| **Week 10** | **16 km** long, slow run run 10 min/ walk 1 min | off | **5 km** steady run | **7 hills** 85% effort 3 km warm-up 3 km cool-down | **7 km** steady run | off | **5 km** steady easy run |
| **Week 11** | **16 km** long, slow run run 10 min/ walk 1 min | off | **5 km** steady run | **8 hills** 85% effort 3 km warm-up 3 km cool-down | **7 km** steady run | off | **6 km** steady easy run |
| **Week 12** | **12 km** long, slow run run 10 min/ walk 1 min | off | **5 km** steady run | **9 hills** 85% effort 3 km warm-up 3 km cool-down | **8 km** steady run | off | **6 km** steady easy run |
| **Week 13** | **18 km** long, slow run run 10 min/ walk 1 min | off | **6 km** steady run | **6 km** fartlek | **8 km** steady run | off | **6 km** steady easy run |
| **Week 14** | **18 km** long, slow run run 10 min/ walk 1 min | off | **6 km** steady run | **4 km** fartlek | **8 km** steady run | off | **6 km** steady easy run |
| **Week 15** | **20 km** long, slow run run 10 min/ walk 1 min | off | **6 km** steady run | **4 km** fartlek | **8 km** steady run | off | **6 km** steady easy run |
| **Week 16** | **6 km** long, slow run run 10 min/ walk 1 min | off | **10 km** steady run | **6 km** steady run | off | off | **3 km** steady easy run |
| **FINALE!** | **21 km** RACE DAY! | | | | | | |

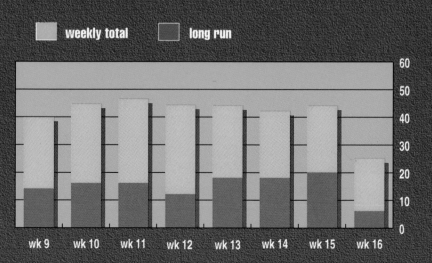

■ weekly total   ■ long run

wk 9 | wk 10 | wk 11 | wk 12 | wk 13 | wk 14 | wk 15 | wk 16

**189**

# To complete a half-marathon
## training program

*miles*

| | SUN | MON | TUES | WED | THURS | FRI | SAT |
|---|---|---|---|---|---|---|---|
| **Week 1** | **4.5 miles** long, slow run run 10 min/ walk 1 min | off | **2.5 miles** steady run | **2 miles** steady run | **2 miles** steady run | off | **2 miles** steady easy run |
| **Week 2** | **4.5 miles** long, slow run run 10 min/ walk 1 min | off | **2.5 miles** steady run | **2 miles** steady run | **2.5 miles** steady run | off | **2 miles** steady easy run |
| **Week 3** | **4.5 miles** long, slow run run 10 min/ walk 1 min | off | **2 miles** steady run | **2.5 miles** steady run | **2 miles** steady run | off | **2.5 miles** steady easy run |
| **Week 4** | **5.5 miles** long, slow run run 10 min/ walk 1 min | off | **2 miles** steady run | **2.5 miles** steady run | **2 miles** steady run | off | **2 miles** steady easy run |
| **Week 5** | **5.5 miles** long, slow run run 10 min/ walk 1 min | off | **2.5 miles** steady run | **2 miles** steady run | **2.5 miles** steady run | off | **2 miles** steady easy run |
| **Week 6** | **6 miles** long, slow run run 10 min/ walk 1 min | off | **2.5 miles** steady run | **3 hills** 85% effort 2 mi warm-up 2 mi cool-down | **3 miles** steady run | off | **2 miles** steady easy run |
| **Week 7** | **6 miles** long, slow run run 10 min/ walk 1 min | off | **2.5 miles** steady run | **4 hills** 85% effort 2 mi warm-up 2 mi cool-down | **3 miles** steady run | off | **2.5 miles** steady easy run |
| **Week 8** | **7.5 miles** long, slow run run 10 min/ walk 1 min | off | **2.5 miles** steady run | **5 hills** 85% effort 2 mi warm-up 2 mi cool-down | **4 miles** steady run | off | **2.5 miles** steady easy run |

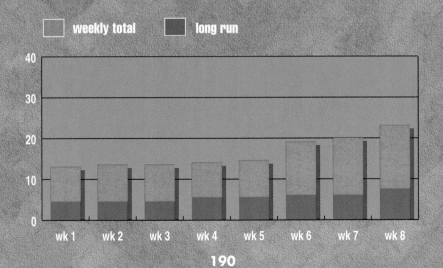

weekly total    long run

190

# *miles*

## To complete a half-marathon
*training program*

| | SUN | MON | TUES | WED | THURS | FRI | SAT |
|---|---|---|---|---|---|---|---|
| **Week 9** | **9 miles** long, slow run run 10 min/ walk 1 min | off | **2.5 miles** steady run | **6 hills** 85% effort 2 mi warm-up 2 mi cool-down | **4 miles** steady run | off | **3 miles** steady easy run |
| **Week 10** | **10 miles** long, slow run run 10 min/ walk 1 min | off | **3 miles** steady run | **7 hills** 85% effort 2 mi warm-up 2 mi cool-down | **4.5 miles** steady run | off | **3 miles** steady easy run |
| **Week 11** | **10 miles** long, slow run run 10 min/ walk 1 min | off | **3 miles** steady run | **8 hills** 85% effort 2 mi warm-up 2 mi cool-down | **4.5 miles** steady run | off | **4 miles** steady easy run |
| **Week 12** | **7.5 miles** long, slow run run 10 min/ walk 1 min | off | **3 miles** steady run | **9 hills** 85% effort 2 mi warm-up 2 mi cool-down | **5 miles** steady run | off | **4 miles** steady easy run |
| **Week 13** | **11 miles** long, slow run run 10 min/ walk 1 min | off | **4 miles** steady run | **4 miles** fartlek | **5 miles** steady run | off | **4 miles** steady easy run |
| **Week 14** | **11 miles** long, slow run run 10 min/ walk 1 min | off | **4 miles** steady run | **2.5 miles** fartlek | **5 miles** steady run | off | **4 miles** steady easy run |
| **Week 15** | **12.5 miles** long, slow run run 10 min/ walk 1 min | off | **4 miles** steady run | **2.5 miles** fartlek | **5 miles** steady run | off | **4 miles** steady easy run |
| **Week 16** | **4 miles** easy run | off | **6 miles** steady run | **4 miles** steady run | off | off | **1.5 miles** easy run |
| **FINALE!** | **13 miles** RACE DAY! | | | | | | |

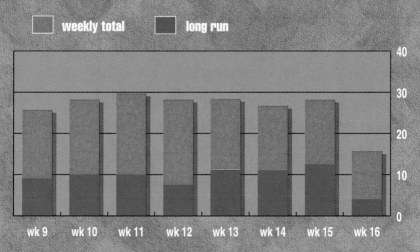

□ weekly total     □ long run

wk 9 | wk 10 | wk 11 | wk 12 | wk 13 | wk 14 | wk 15 | wk 16

# 2 hr. half-marathon
*training program*

**kilometres**

| | SUN | MON | TUES | WED | THURS | FRI | SAT |
|---|---|---|---|---|---|---|---|
| **Week 1** | 7 km<br>run 10 min/<br>walk 1 min<br>6:15–6:30 pace | off | 4 km<br>steady run<br>5:55 pace | 3 km<br>steady run<br>5:55 pace | 3 km<br>steady run<br>5:55 pace | off | 3 km<br>steady<br>easy run |
| **Week 2** | 7 km<br>run 10 min/<br>walk 1 min<br>6:15–6:30 pace | off | 4 km<br>steady run<br>5:55 pace | 3 km<br>steady run<br>5:55 pace | 4 km<br>steady run<br>5:55 pace | off | 3 km<br>steady<br>easy run |
| **Week 3** | 7 km<br>run 10 min/<br>walk 1 min<br>6:15–6:30 pace | off | 3 km<br>steady run<br>5:55 pace | 4 km<br>steady run<br>5:55 pace | 3 km<br>steady run<br>5:55 pace | off | 4 km<br>steady<br>easy run |
| **Week 4** | 9 km<br>run 10 min/<br>walk 1 min<br>6:15–6:30 pace | off | 4 km<br>steady run<br>5:55 pace | 4 km<br>steady run<br>5:55 pace | 3 km<br>steady run<br>5:55 pace | off | 3 km<br>steady<br>easy run |
| **Week 5** | 9 km<br>run 10 min/<br>walk 1 min<br>6:15–6:30 pace | off | 5 km<br>steady run<br>5:55 pace | 3 km<br>steady run<br>5:55 pace | 4 km<br>steady run<br>5:55 pace | off | 3 km<br>steady<br>easy run |
| **Week 6** | 10 km<br>run 10 min/<br>walk 1 min<br>6:15–6:30 pace | off | 4 km<br>steady run<br>5:55 pace | 3 hills<br>85% effort<br>3 km warm-up<br>3 km cool-down | 5 km<br>steady run<br>5:55 pace | off | 3 km<br>steady<br>easy run |
| **Week 7** | 10 km<br>run 10 min/<br>walk 1 min<br>6:15–6:30 pace | off | 4 km<br>steady run<br>5:55 pace | 4 hills<br>85% effort<br>3 km warm-up<br>3 km cool-down | 5 km<br>steady run<br>5:55 pace | off | 4 km<br>steady<br>easy run |
| **Week 8** | 12 km<br>run 10 min/<br>walk 1 min<br>6:15–6:30 pace | off | 4 km<br>steady run<br>5:55 pace | 5 hills<br>85% effort<br>3 km warm-up<br>3 km cool-down | 6 km<br>steady run<br>5:55 pace | off | 4 km<br>steady<br>easy run |

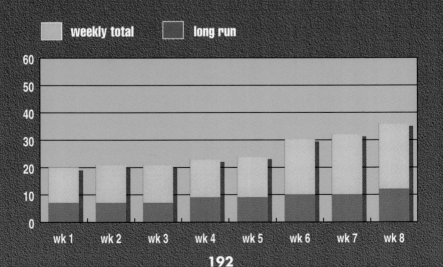

weekly total   long run

# kilometres

# 2 hr. half-marathon
## *training program*

| | SUN | MON | TUES | WED | THURS | FRI | SAT |
|---|---|---|---|---|---|---|---|
| **Week 9** | **14 km** run 10 min/ walk 1 min 6:15–6:30 pace | off | **4 km** steady run 5:55 pace | **6 hills** 85% effort 3 km warm-up 3 km cool-down | **6 km** steady run 5:55 pace | off | **5 km** steady easy run |
| **Week 10** | **16 km** run 10 min/ walk 1 min 6:15–6:30 pace | off | **5 km** steady run 5:55 pace | **7 hills** 85% effort 3 km warm-up 3 km cool-down | **7 km** steady run 5:55 pace | off | **5 km** steady easy run |
| **Week 11** | **16 km** run 10 min/ walk 1 min 6:15–6:30 pace | off | **5 km** steady run 5:55 pace | **8 hills** 85% effort 3 km warm-up 3 km cool-down | **7 km** steady run 5:55 pace | off | **6 km** steady easy run |
| **Week 12** | **12 km** run 10 min/ walk 1 min 6:15–6:30 pace | off | **5 km** steady run 5:55 pace | **9 hills** 85% effort 3 km warm-up 3 km cool-down | **8 km** steady run 5:55 pace | off | **6 km** steady easy run |
| **Week 13** | **18 km** run 10 min/ walk 1 min 6:15–6:30 pace | off | **6 km** steady run 5:55 pace | **2 speed int.** 1.6 km @ 4:50/km 3 km warm-up 3 km cool-down | **8 km** steady run 5:55 pace | off | **6 km** steady easy run |
| **Week 14** | **18 km** run 10 min/ walk 1 min 6:15–6:30 pace | off | **6 km** steady run 5:55 pace | **3 speed int.** 1.6 km @ 4:50/km 3 km warm-up 3 km cool-down | **8 km** steady run 5:55 pace | off | **6 km** steady easy run |
| **Week 15** | **20 km** run 10 min/ walk 1 min 6:15–6:30 pace | off | **6 km** steady run 5:55 pace | **4 speed int.** 1.6 km @ 4:50/km 3 km warm-up 3 km cool-down | **8 km** steady run 5:55 pace | off | **6 km** steady easy run |
| **Week 16** | **6 km** steady run 5:55 pace | off | **10 km** steady run 5:55 pace | **6 km** steady run 5:55 pace | off | off | **3 km** steady easy run |
| **FINALE!** | **21 km** RACE DAY! 5:41 pace | | | | | | |

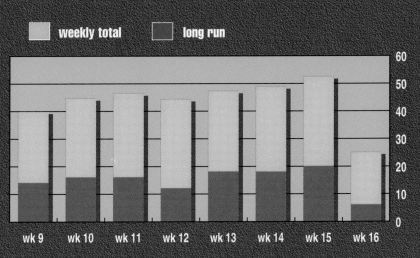

weekly total ▢  long run ▢

wk 9 | wk 10 | wk 11 | wk 12 | wk 13 | wk 14 | wk 15 | wk 16

**193**

# 2 hr. half-marathon
*training program*

miles

| | SUN | MON | TUES | WED | THURS | FRI | SAT |
|---|---|---|---|---|---|---|---|
| **Week 1** | **4.5 miles**<br>run 10 min/<br>walk 1 min<br>9:45–10:15 pace | off | **2.5 miles**<br>steady run<br>9:30 pace | **2 miles**<br>steady run<br>9:30 pace | **2 miles**<br>steady run<br>9:30 pace | off | **2 miles**<br>steady<br>easy run |
| **Week 2** | **4.5 miles**<br>run 10 min/<br>walk 1 min<br>9:45–10:15 pace | off | **2.5 miles**<br>steady run<br>9:30 pace | **2 miles**<br>steady run<br>9:30 pace | **2.5 miles**<br>steady run<br>9:30 pace | off | **2 miles**<br>steady<br>easy run |
| **Week 3** | **4.5 miles**<br>run 10 min/<br>walk 1 min<br>9:45–10:15 pace | off | **2 miles**<br>steady run<br>9:30 pace | **2.5 miles**<br>steady run<br>9:30 pace | **2 miles**<br>steady run<br>9:30 pace | off | **2.5 miles**<br>steady<br>easy run |
| **Week 4** | **5.5 miles**<br>run 10 min/<br>walk 1 min<br>9:45–10:15 pace | off | **2 miles**<br>steady run<br>9:30 pace | **2.5 miles**<br>steady run<br>9:30 pace | **2 miles**<br>steady run<br>9:30 pace | off | **2 miles**<br>steady<br>easy run |
| **Week 5** | **5.5 miles**<br>run 10 min/<br>walk 1 min<br>9:45–10:15 pace | off | **3 miles**<br>steady run<br>9:30 pace | **2 miles**<br>steady run<br>9:30 pace | **2.5 miles**<br>steady run<br>9:30 pace | off | **2 miles**<br>steady<br>easy run |
| **Week 6** | **6 miles**<br>run 10 min/<br>walk 1 min<br>9:45–10:15 pace | off | **2.5 miles**<br>steady run<br>9:30 pace | **3 hills**<br>85% effort<br>2 mi warm-up<br>2 mi cool-down | **3 miles**<br>steady run<br>9:30 pace | off | **2 miles**<br>steady<br>easy run |
| **Week 7** | **6 miles**<br>run 10 min/<br>walk 1 min<br>9:45–10:15 pace | off | **2.5 miles**<br>steady run<br>9:30 pace | **4 hills**<br>85% effort<br>2 mi warm-up<br>2 mi cool-down | **3 miles**<br>steady run<br>9:30 pace | off | **2.5 miles**<br>steady<br>easy run |
| **Week 8** | **7.5 miles**<br>run 10 min/<br>walk 1 min<br>9:45–10:15 pace | off | **2.5 miles**<br>steady run<br>9:30 pace | **5 hills**<br>85% effort<br>2 mi warm-up<br>2 mi cool-down | **4 miles**<br>steady run<br>9:30 pace | off | **2.5 miles**<br>steady<br>easy run |

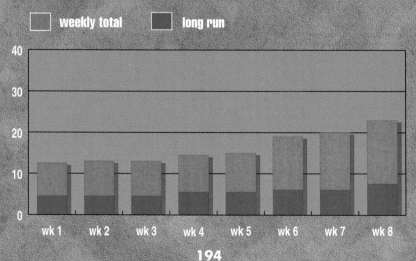

□ weekly total   □ long run

# 2 hr. half-marathon
*training program*

| | SUN | MON | TUES | WED | THURS | FRI | SAT |
|---|---|---|---|---|---|---|---|
| **Week 9** | **9 miles** run 10 min/ walk 1 min 9:45–10:15 pace | off | **2.5 miles** steady run 9:30 pace | **6 hills** 85% effort 2 mi warm-up 2 mi cool-down | **4 miles** steady run 9:30 pace | off | **3 miles** steady easy run |
| **Week 10** | **10 miles** run 10 min/ walk 1 min 9:45–10:15 pace | off | **3 miles** steady run 9:30 pace | **7 hills** 85% effort 2 mi warm-up 2 mi cool-down | **4.5 miles** steady run 9:30 pace | off | **3 miles** steady easy run |
| **Week 11** | **10 miles** run 10 min/ walk 1 min 9:45–10:15 pace | off | **3 miles** steady run 9:30 pace | **8 hills** 85% effort 2 mi warm-up 2 mi cool-down | **4.5 miles** steady run 9:30 pace | off | **4 miles** steady easy run |
| **Week 12** | **7.5 miles** run 10 min/ walk 1 min 9:45–10:15 pace | off | **3 miles** steady run 9:30 pace | **9 hills** 85% effort 2 mi warm-up 2 mi cool-down | **5 miles** steady run 9:30 pace | off | **4 miles** steady easy run |
| **Week 13** | **11 miles** run 10 min/ walk 1 min 9:45–10:15 pace | off | **4 miles** steady run 9:30 pace | **2 speed int.** 1 mi @ 7:45/mi 2 mi warm-up 2 mi cool-down | **5 miles** steady run 9:30 pace | off | **4 miles** steady easy run |
| **Week 14** | **11 miles** run 10 min/ walk 1 min 9:45–10:15 pace | off | **4 miles** steady run 9:30 pace | **3 speed int.** 1 mi @ 7:45/mi 2 mi warm-up 2 mi cool-down | **5 miles** steady run 9:30 pace | off | **4 miles** steady easy run |
| **Week 15** | **12.5 miles** run 10 min/ walk 1 min 9:45–10:15 pace | off | **4 miles** steady run 9:30 pace | **4 speed int.** 1 mi @ 7:45/mi 2 mi warm-up 2 mi cool-down | **5 miles** steady run 9:30 pace | off | **4 miles** steady easy run |
| **Week 16** | **4 miles** easy run 9:30 pace | off | **6 miles** steady run 9:30 pace | **4 miles** steady run 9:30 pace | off | off | **2 miles** easy run |
| **FINALE!** | **13 miles** RACE DAY! 9:09 pace | | | | | | |

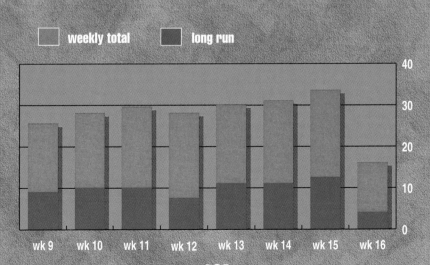

□ weekly total    □ long run

# 1 hr. 40 min. half-marathon
*training program*

## kilometres

| | SUN | MON | TUES | WED | THURS | FRI | SAT |
|---|---|---|---|---|---|---|---|
| **Week 1** | 7 km steady run 5:15–5:30 pace | off | 4 km steady run 5:00 pace | 3 km steady run easy run | 3 km steady run 5:00–5:15 pace | off | 3 km steady easy run |
| **Week 2** | 7 km steady run 5:15–5:30 pace | off | 4 km steady run 5:00 pace | 3 km steady run easy run | 4 km steady run 5:00–5:15 pace | off | 3 km steady easy run |
| **Week 3** | 7 km steady run 5:15–5:30 pace | off | 3 km steady run 5:00 pace | 4 km steady run easy run | 3 km steady run 5:00–5:15 pace | off | 4 km steady easy run |
| **Week 4** | 9 km steady run 5:15–5:30 pace | off | 4 km steady run 5:00 pace | 4 km steady run easy run | 3 km steady run 5:00–5:15 pace | off | 3 km steady easy run |
| **Week 5** | 9 km steady run 5:15–5:30 pace | off | 5 km steady run 5:00 pace | 3 km steady run easy run | 4 km steady run 5:00–5:15 pace | off | 3 km steady easy run |
| **Week 6** | 10 km steady run 5:15–5:30 pace | off | 4 km steady run 5:00 pace | 3 hills 85% effort 3 km warm-up 3 km cool-down | 5 km steady run 5:00–5:15 pace | off | 4 km steady easy run |
| **Week 7** | 10 km steady run 5:15–5:30 pace | off | 4 km steady run 5:00 pace | 4 hills 85% effort 3 km warm-up 3 km cool-down | 5 km steady run 5:00–5:15 pace | off | 4 km steady easy run |
| **Week 8** | 12 km steady run 5:15–5:30 pace | off | 4 km steady run 5:00 pace | 5 hills 85% effort 3 km warm-up 3 km cool-down | 6 km steady run 5:00–5:15 pace | off | 4 km steady easy run |

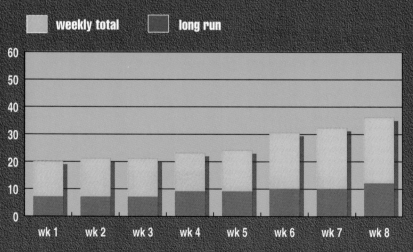

weekly total    long run

196

# kilometres

## 1 hr. 40 min. half-marathon
### training program

| | SUN | MON | TUES | WED | THURS | FRI | SAT |
|---|---|---|---|---|---|---|---|
| **Week 9** | **14 km** steady run 5:15–5:30 pace | off | **4 km** steady run 5:00 pace | **6 hills** 85% effort 3 km warm-up 3 km cool-down | **6 km** steady run 5:00–5:15 pace | off | **5 km** steady easy run |
| **Week 10** | **16 km** steady run 5:15–5:30 pace | off | **5 km** fartlek 4:45–5:30 pace | **7 hills** 85% effort 3 km warm-up 3 km cool-down | **7 km** steady run 5:00–5:15 pace | off | **5 km** steady easy run |
| **Week 11** | **16 km** steady run 5:15–5:30 pace | off | **5 km** fartlek 4:45–5:30 pace | **8 hills** 85% effort 3 km warm-up 3 km cool-down | **7 km** steady run 5:00–5:15 pace | off | **6 km** steady easy run |
| **Week 12** | **12 km** steady run 5:15–5:30 pace | off | **5 km** fartlek 4:45–5:30 pace | **9 hills** 85% effort 3 km warm-up 3 km cool-down | **8 km** steady run 5:00–5:15 pace | off | **6 km** steady easy run |
| **Week 13** | **18 km** steady run 5:15–5:30 pace | off | **6 km** fartlek 4:45–5:30 pace | **2 speed int.** 1.6 km @ 4:10/km 3 km warm-up 3 km cool-down | **8 km** steady run 5:00–5:15 pace | off | **6 km** steady easy run |
| **Week 14** | **18 km** steady run 5:15–5:30 pace | off | **6 km** fartlek 4:45–5:30 pace | **3 speed int.** 1.6 km @ 4:10/km 3 km warm-up 3 km cool-down | **8 km** steady run 5:00–5:15 pace | off | **6 km** steady easy run |
| **Week 15** | **20 km** steady run 5:15–5:30 pace | off | **6 km** fartlek 4:45–5:30 pace | **4 speed int.** 1.6 km @ 4:10/km 3 km warm-up 3 km cool-down | **8 km** steady run 5:00–5:15 pace | off | **6 km** steady easy run |
| **Week 16** | **6 km** steady run 5:00 pace | off | **10 km** steady run 5:00 pace | **6 km** steady run 5:00 pace | off | off | **3 km** easy run |
| **FINALE!** | **21 km** RACE DAY! 4:44 pace | | | | | | |

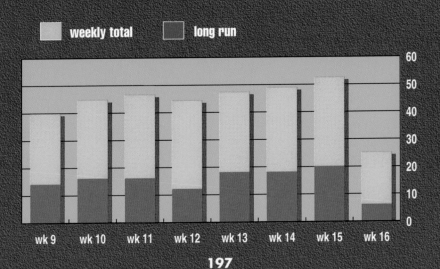

weekly total    long run

60
50
40
30
20
10
0

wk 9   wk 10   wk 11   wk 12   wk 13   wk 14   wk 15   wk 16

# 1 hr. 40 min. half-marathon
## training program

| | SUN | MON | TUES | WED | THURS | FRI | SAT |
|---|---|---|---|---|---|---|---|
| **Week 1** | 4.5 miles<br>steady run<br>8:30–9:00 pace | off | 2.5 miles<br>steady run<br>8:00 pace | 2 miles<br>steady<br>easy run | 2 miles<br>steady run<br>8:00–8:30 pace | off | 2 miles<br>steady<br>easy run |
| **Week 2** | 4.5 miles<br>steady run<br>8:30–9:00 pace | off | 2.5 miles<br>steady run<br>8:00 pace | 2 miles<br>steady<br>easy run | 2.5 miles<br>steady run<br>8:00–8:30 pace | off | 2 miles<br>steady<br>easy run |
| **Week 3** | 4.5 miles<br>steady run<br>8:30–9:00 pace | off | 2 miles<br>steady run<br>8:00 pace | 2.5 miles<br>steady<br>easy run | 2 miles<br>steady run<br>8:00–8:30 pace | off | 2.5 miles<br>steady<br>easy run |
| **Week 4** | 5.5 miles<br>steady run<br>8:30–9:00 pace | off | 2.5 miles<br>steady run<br>8:00 pace | 2.5 miles<br>steady<br>easy run | 2 miles<br>steady run<br>8:00–8:30 pace | off | 2 miles<br>steady<br>easy run |
| **Week 5** | 5.5 miles<br>steady run<br>8:30–9:00 pace | off | 3 miles<br>steady run<br>8:00 pace | 2 miles<br>steady<br>easy run | 2.5 miles<br>steady run<br>8:00–8:30 pace | off | 2 miles<br>steady<br>easy run |
| **Week 6** | 6 miles<br>steady run<br>8:30–9:00 pace | off | 2.5 miles<br>steady run<br>8:00 pace | 3 hills<br>85% effort<br>2 mi warm-up<br>2 mi cool-down | 3 miles<br>steady run<br>8:00–8:30 pace | off | 2.5 miles<br>steady<br>easy run |
| **Week 7** | 6 miles<br>steady run<br>8:30–9:00 pace | off | 2.5 miles<br>steady run<br>8:00 pace | 4 hills<br>85% effort<br>2 mi warm-up<br>2 mi cool-down | 3 miles<br>steady run<br>8:00–8:30 pace | off | 2.5 miles<br>steady<br>easy run |
| **Week 8** | 7.5 miles<br>steady run<br>8:30–9:00 pace | off | 2.5 miles<br>steady run<br>8:00 pace | 5 hills<br>85% effort<br>2 mi warm-up<br>2 mi cool-down | 4 miles<br>steady run<br>8:00–8:30 pace | off | 2.5 miles<br>steady<br>easy run |

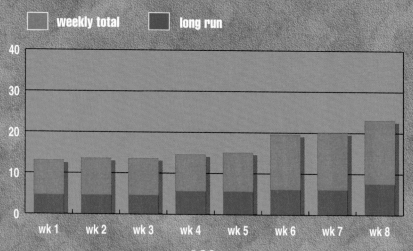

☐ weekly total     ☐ long run

# *miles*

| | SUN | MON | TUES | WED | THURS | FRI | SAT |
|---|---|---|---|---|---|---|---|
| **Week 9** | **9 miles**<br>steady run<br>8:30–9:00 pace | off | **2.5 miles**<br>steady run<br>8:00 pace | **6 hills**<br>85% effort<br>2 mi warm-up<br>2 mi cool-down | **4 miles**<br>steady run<br>8:00–8:30 pace | off | **3 miles**<br>steady<br>easy run |
| **Week 10** | **10 miles**<br>steady run<br>8:30–9:00 pace | off | **3 miles**<br>fartlek<br>7:40–8:50 pace | **7 hills**<br>85% effort<br>2 mi warm-up<br>2 mi cool-down | **4.5 miles**<br>steady run<br>8:00–8:30 pace | off | **3 miles**<br>steady<br>easy run |
| **Week 11** | **10 miles**<br>steady run<br>8:30–9:00 pace | off | **3 miles**<br>fartlek<br>7:40–8:50 pace | **8 hills**<br>85% effort<br>2 mi warm-up<br>2 mi cool-down | **4.5 miles**<br>steady run<br>8:00–8:30 pace | off | **4 miles**<br>steady<br>easy run |
| **Week 12** | **7.5 miles**<br>steady run<br>8:30–9:00 pace | off | **3 miles**<br>fartlek<br>7:40–8:50 pace | **9 hills**<br>85% effort<br>2 mi warm-up<br>2 mi cool-down | **5 miles**<br>steady run<br>8:00–8:30 pace | off | **4 miles**<br>steady<br>easy run |
| **Week 13** | **11 miles**<br>steady run<br>8:30–9:00 pace | off | **4 miles**<br>fartlek<br>7:40–8:50 pace | **2 speed int.**<br>1 mi @ 6:45/mi<br>2 mi warm-up<br>2 mi cool-down | **5 miles**<br>steady run<br>8:00–8:30 pace | off | **4 miles**<br>steady<br>easy run |
| **Week 14** | **11 miles**<br>steady run<br>8:30–9:00 pace | off | **4 miles**<br>fartlek<br>7:40–8:50 pace | **3 speed int.**<br>1 mi @ 6:45/mi<br>2 mi warm-up<br>2 mi cool-down | **5 miles**<br>steady run<br>8:00–8:30 pace | off | **4 miles**<br>steady<br>easy run |
| **Week 15** | **12.5 miles**<br>steady run<br>8:30–9:00 pace | off | **4 miles**<br>fartlek<br>7:40–8:50 pace | **4 speed int.**<br>1 mi @ 6:45/mi<br>2 mi warm-up<br>2 mi cool-down | **5 miles**<br>steady run<br>8:00–8:30 pace | off | **4 miles**<br>steady<br>easy run |
| **Week 16** | **4 miles**<br>easy run<br>8:00 pace | off | **6 miles**<br>steady run<br>8:00 pace | **4 miles**<br>steady run<br>8:00 pace | off | off | **2 miles**<br>easy run |
| **FINALE!** | **13 miles**<br>RACE DAY!<br>7:38 pace | | | | | | |

☐ weekly total   ☐ long run

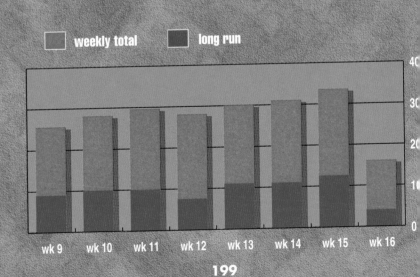

| | | | | | | | |
|---|---|---|---|---|---|---|---|
| wk 9 | wk 10 | wk 11 | wk 12 | wk 13 | wk 14 | wk 15 | wk 16 |

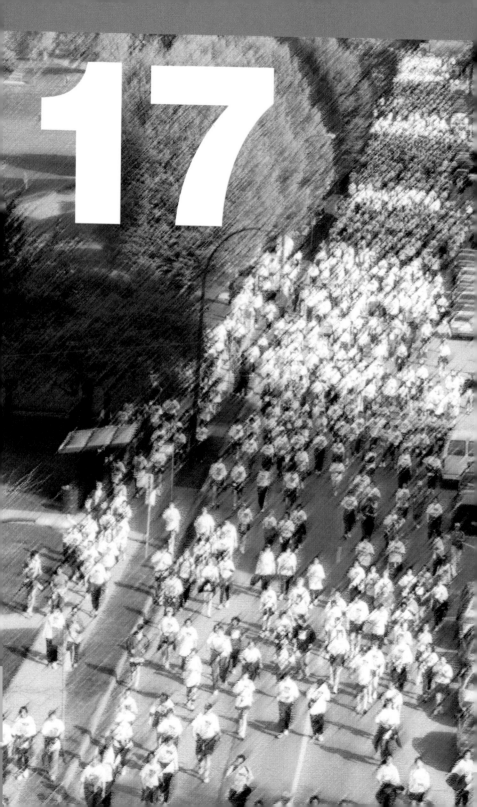

17

# The Marathon

Are you ready for the ultimate running challenge? You'll find it in the marathon.

Training for the marathon can positively change the way you look at the rest of your life: you will experience a dramatic change in your physical and mental outlook on life and you will gain the self-confidence to achieve both your athletic and personal goals. By training to run a marathon, you'll find personal resources you didn't know were there.

The largest-growing group in the modern marathon is composed of people who just want to complete the 26.2-mile (42-km) course. Over the years it has become obvious that not all of us can be competitive marathoners: just as our fingerprints are unique to each of us, so are our other attributes, such as body type, resting heart rate, maximum heart rate and requirements put on us by family, work, friends and commitments to the community.

If you decide the marathon is your event, don't plan on doing more than two in a year. This gives you lots of time to rest, recover and start training for the next race.

## Hitting the Wall

The biggest problem runners usually have to contend with during the marathon is "hitting the wall," a catchy phrase for depleting the glycogen stores in their muscles. Much of your success in the marathon will depend on energy conservation and efficient fuel utilization. If your glycogen runs out, the race is over, whether you have reached the finish line or not.

Long slow training runs teach your body how to use its fuel more efficiently, and they promote the utilization of fat (you probably have enough to run dozens of marathons), which conserves glycogen. With proper long training runs, the "wall" will move farther and farther away, until finally it does not appear at all during the marathon.

People often ask why it is necessary to do the weekly long runs at such an agonizingly slow pace. Quite simply, you are running them for endurance, not speed, and if you train too fast, you will not only be too tired to benefit from your other runs that week, you will also greatly increase your risk of injury.

CH. 17

First-time marathoners should take a walking break of 1 minute for every 10 minutes of running on their long runs (and during the race itself). These walking breaks will only slow you down by about 15 seconds a mile (9 seconds a kilometre), which is less than 7 minutes for the entire marathon. By not taking these short breaks, especially at the beginning, you may end up going slower rather than faster because of the accumulated fatigue.

Experienced marathoners should be running their long runs at 1 to 1$^1$/$_2$ minutes a mile ($^1$/$_2$ to 1 minute a kilometre) slower than their planned race pace. Everyone should be able to pass the talk test, which means you should be able to carry on a conversation without gasping for breath. If you can't talk, you're running too fast.

## Where is the wall?

- **It starts at the length of your longest continuous run in the last two to three weeks.**

- **You can bring it closer by running too fast**

- **You can move it farther away it by running slower or inserting 1-minute walking breaks every 10 minutes.**

# Tapering

Many experienced marathoners will tell you that you'll only perform as well as you've tapered. Many people forget that training is hard work and you can't just jump into an event and perform well without proper planning. Everyone's performance can benefit from a good taper, which is a carefully planned period of reduced training. This gradual easing up allows your body to disperse the residual fatigue products that have been carried from one workout to another. The extra recovery and regeneration that can occur during a taper result in what is called peaking. Come race day, your legs will have that extra snap to ensure your best performance.

The biggest complaint I get about tapering is that people often feel extremely restless during this period—they feel like they should be doing more. Don't. The beginning of the taper period signifies the end of training—and the beginning of competition preparation—and any hard training done during this period will do more to hurt your performance than help it because you won't recover fast enough. A good taper will make you feel like a horse in the gaits at the start of the Belmont for the few days before your event. It is the feeling of peak fitness; use it to your advantage.

CH. 17

A taper for a marathon should generally take up the last two to three weeks before the event—your last long run should take place no later than two weeks before the event. During the taper period, you should run only 30 to 50 percent of your regular weekly distance. The best tapers have runners maintaining their training intensity while gradually reducing their training distance to practically zero a few days before the event. Focus on keeping the intensity up on your continuous runs and reducing their length significantly. Forget speed training if you have any planned.

Your last quality workout should be on the Sunday before the race. Run 10 miles (16 km) at your target pace for the marathon. This run is a high-quality workout that requires your discipline, so it is best to run it alone and concentrate on your form and setting your targeted pace. Do not race or get in a race with one of your training partners.

Starting on Monday, you will begin to cut back your distance in the tapering phase of the program. Some people feel very heavy and their disposition suffers during the tapering phase. Concentrate on the joy of less distance and the fact that you have all this extra time to relax and enjoy the tapering phase.

The most important day is two days prior to the race. Take the day off, go to bed early and enjoy as much sleep as possible. Stay in bed, read and relax. Even if you can't sleep, stay lying down—it's the best way to get you ready for race day. Remember, nothing you do in the final week will help you, but everything you do can hinder your performance. Quality training takes at least two weeks to improve your performance, but overtraining can affect your performance the next day.

Visualization is a key part of the week as you relax and think about your training and the goals you have set for the marathon. Read or listen to some of your favourite music to motivate yourself.

# Race Day Tips

## Rule #1: Relax!

The most important advice we can give to the first-time racer is to relax. Enjoy yourself; racing is meant to be a stimulating, memorable experience that helps keep things in proper perspective. Your goal is simply to finish. Your first marathon is for the experience, not for the competition, so don't try to break any records. Even if something goes wrong on your first race—say you get stomach cramps or your shoelaces come untied—it's not the end of the world. You'll live to run and race again.

CH. 17

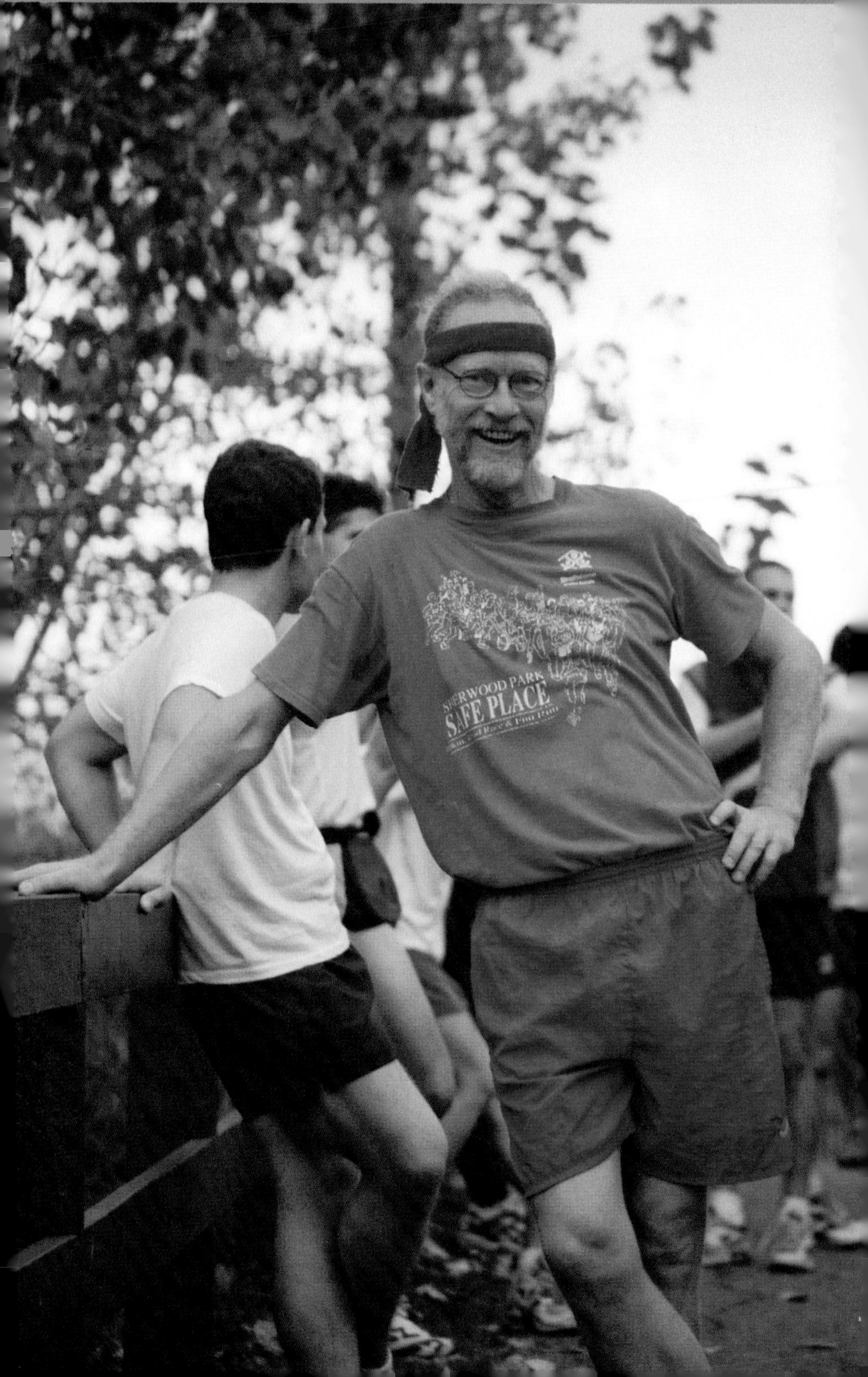
SHERWOOD PARK
SAFE PLACE

# Eating and drinking

Don't eat or drink anything out of the ordinary. The day of a race is no time to experiment, no matter what you may have heard about athletic super-foods. Don't be concerned about the carbohydrate loading that you've heard is favoured by marathon runners, either. In fact, for your last meal (eaten at least 3 hours before race time) you might want to eat less than normal, because nervousness could upset your digestive system.

If it's an early start—many marathons start very early to avoid the heat of the day—try eating a nutritional energy bar or a bowl of instant oatmeal for breakfast about $1^1/_2$ hours before race time. These easily digestible, high-carbohydrate foods won't challenge your digestive system. Also, they are easy to pack and eat in a hotel room if you travelled to the race.

In warm weather, drink a full cup of water before the start of the race. Continue drinking every mile or two during the race. You should practise the same on hot-weather training runs. Don't ever forget: heat can kill. Adjust your expectations—don't try to be a hero—and drink fluids at every opportunity.

# Strategy

Planning your race strategy in advance will build your confidence. Break the course into small sections, making sure you know where hills and other key landmarks are located. It's particularly important that you know the last 800 metres of the course—run it as a warm-up on race day, and set a few landmarks in your mind.

# Getting ready

When you arrive at the race, don't be intimidated by what you see other runners doing. Many of them are preparing for a hard effort, whereas you want to make sure you save your energy for a more comfortable race. Do some walking, some stretching and some light jogging to loosen up.

# Lining up and starting

Make your way to the back of the starting pack where you won't get caught in the starting sprint. Begin slowly. Don't worry about all the runners who take off ahead of you. It's far better to start slowly and catch up later than to begin too fast and be passed by hundreds of runners after a mile or two. Once you get room to run freely, move into your normal, relaxed training pace. Maintain that pace (it should be one that allows you to talk comfortably) at least until you reach the halfway mark. Then, if you feel strong and want to pick it up, go ahead—but make sure you do it gradually. If you reach a point of struggle, slow down to recover your strength.

CH. 17

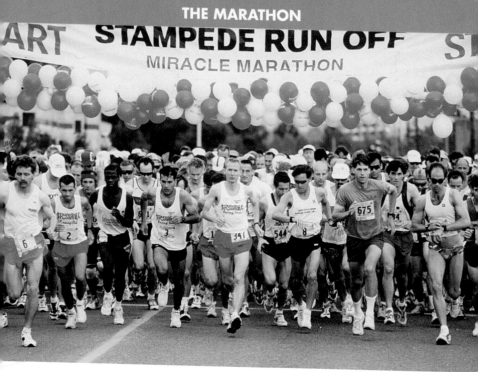

## Walking

Nowhere on the entry blank does it say that you can't walk, so if you feel the need, take walking breaks, particularly on the hills. Never stop moving forwards, however, unless you are hurt. There's a nice way to "cheat" a little and disguise your walking breaks: because drinking water is so important during a race, many runners stop and drink when they get to the water tables. You can do the same—getting water plus the walking rest you need—and no one will be the wiser.

## Finishing

Don't finish with a sprint. It is not only unwise, but it can be dangerous. Concentrate on finishing with a good, relaxed, strong form.

## Recovery

After you finish, be sure you walk around for a cool-down. Drink plenty of fluids, especially if it's a hot day. Change into dry clothes as soon as possible, and when you get home, stretch your muscles thoroughly after taking a warm bath. Don't do any running the next day, although it's OK to swim or bike. You might find it hard to contain your newfound racing enthusiasm, but to run on leg muscles that might be sore would only tempt injury. You should probably

CH. 17

plan on resting completely for the next week, which means light jogging at the most. Once that heavy-leg feeling dissipates, start easing back into running. One rule of thumb is to take one day of rest for each mile raced—that means no racing, hard running, speed work or hill training for 26 days after the marathon. Rest is important. Your hard-earned base is still there, and you will be back at a higher level of fitness if you take the time to rest.

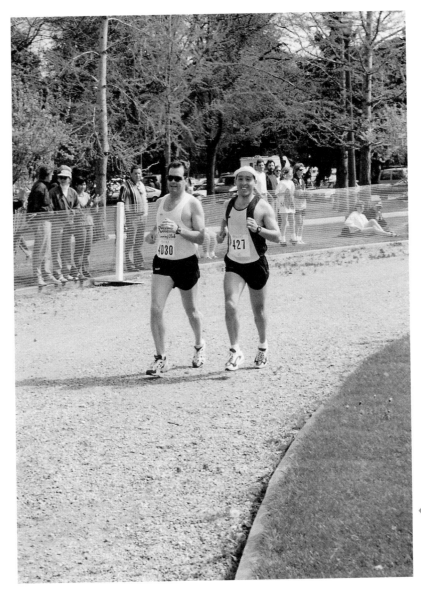

CH. 1

## Systems Review

**Principles**
- Relaxation.
- Efficiency of form.
- Economy of effort and motion.
- Staying within yourself.
- Maintaining a positive attitude.
- Staying with a successful program.

**Pacing**
- Stay within yourself.
- For the first 5 miles (8 km), your mile pace should be about 10 seconds slower than average.
- Your mile pace during the first half should average 2 to 3 seconds slower than during the second half.
- Brisk walk at all of the water stations in the first half of the race.

**Striding**
- Don't over-stride!
- Keep your stride short going uphill.
- Avoid the temptation to over-stride going downhill.
- As you tire, concentrate on a shorter stride and quicker turnover.

**Be Positive**
- Everyone gets negative messages. Only those who listen slow dramatically.
- Have a strategy for projecting positive thoughts to confront the negative.
- Words or phrases relating to past successes will bring future success.
- Learn how to shift into the right brain.

**Have Fun!**
- If you enjoy this run, you'll want to do it again and you'll get better.
- Talk to people, share stories, enjoy the course.

# Marathon Training Questions

## How can I race 26 miles when my long run is only 20 miles?

Over the years, there have been a variety of training programs that over-extend the long run beyond the marathon distance. My experience is that the frequency of injury increases as we extend the long run beyond the 20-mile (32-km) distance. I have seen too many folks run a great long run of 25 to 28 miles (40 to 45 km) and then on marathon day come up with a disappointing time. The reason is that they did not give themselves enough time to recover from the long extended run.

Your training program is made up of base training, strength training and speed training. You train specifically in each phase; then on race day you put it all together and run the marathon. Your distances should be looked at over a four-week period, not on one individual day. The taper phase of your training allows you to rest and recover from training and then perform to a higher standard on race day.

Another key ingredient on race day is your adrenaline level, which, together with the group support and the crowd, can carry you for that extra distance.

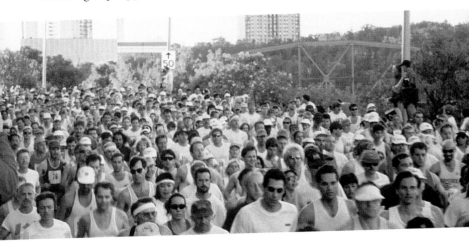

## How can I run my targeted pace in the marathon when I have run my long training runs slower?

Slowing the long runs down helps you recover faster, still gives you the desired endurance training effect and dramatically lowers your injury risk. You have plenty of hills, intervals and fartlek sessions to run at race pace or faster to give you the speed. If you ran your long runs at nearly race pace, you would need one day per mile to recover—it would take you 20 days to recover from a 20-mile (32-km) training run. By slowing your pace by 15 to 20 percent, you will find that within a day or two you are ready to train hard, allowing you to do quality strength or speed work. This approach is called specific training.

## How can I prevent injury and be sure I make it to the start line?

Many talented runners who approach their training in an overzealous manner end up sidelined by injury. Keep your training fun, keep it specific, keep it to the program and do not add to the program. Your training program is planned so that you will continually improve and get stronger. More is not necessarily better—fatigue will rob you of energy, both mentally and physically. Remember, running is playtime; don't make it feel like work!

## How much of my total weekly distance should be speed?

Speed work should account for no more than 8 to 10 percent of your total weekly distance. Stick to the program and don't add any speed to your endurance training sessions. Training faster too often won't give your body enough time to recover between sessions.

# Choosing Your Program

Before you start training for a marathon, you should have a reasonable, intelligent goal for the race. Take a look at the following summaries and choose the level that best suits your needs and abilities. Take all the elements into consideration: your 1-mile pace, the weekly training distance required, the training pace for the long run and the race pace for the marathon.

## To complete the marathon

Race pace: to complete

Long run pace: 10:30 to 11:30 min./mile (6:30 to 7:10 min./km)

1-mile time trial: 8:00 min.

10-K time trial: 60:00 min.

Base training: 25 to 30 miles (40 to 48 km) a week

H. 17

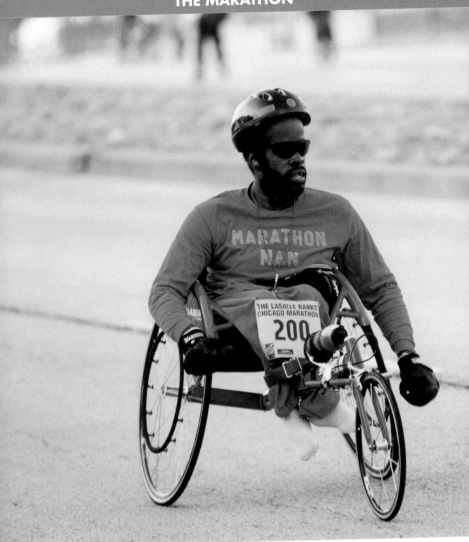

## 4-hour marathon

Race pace: 9:10 min./mile (5:44 min./km)

Long run pace: 9:30 to 10:30 min./mile (5:55 to 6:30 min./km)

1-mile time trial: 7:15 min.

10-K time trial: 50:00 min.

Base training: 30 to 35 miles (48 to 56 km) a week

CH. 1

## 3-hour-45-minute marathon

Race pace: 8:35 min./mile (5:20 min./km)

Long run pace: 8:45 to 10:00 min./mile (5:25 to 6:15 min./km)

1-mile time trial: 6:45 min.

10-K time trial: 47 min.

Base training: 35 to 40 miles (56 to 64 km) a week

## 3-hour-30-minute marathon

Race pace: 7:59 min./mile (4:58 min./km)

Long run pace: 8:30 to 9:30 per mile (5:15 to 5:55 min./km)

1-mile time trial: 6:20 min.

10-K-time trial: 44 min.

Base training: 40 to 45 miles (64 to 72 km) a week

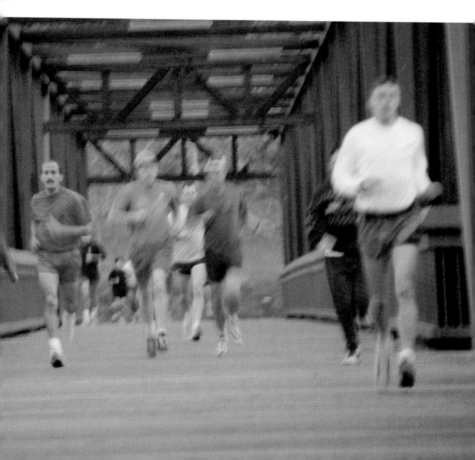

## 3-hour-10-minute marathon

Race pace: 7:14 min./mile (4:30 min./km)

Long run pace: 8:00 to 9:00 min./mile (5:00 to 5:35 min./km)

1-mile time trial: 6:20 min.

10-K time trial: 44 min.

Base training: 40 to 45 miles (64 to 72 km) a week

## Sub-3-hour marathon

Race pace: 6:50 min./mile (4:15 min./km)

Long run pace: 7:30 to 8:30 min./mile (4:40 to 5:15 min./km)

1-mile time trial: 5:35 min.

10-K time trial: 38 min.

Base training: 45 to 60 miles (72 to 96 km) a week

The training schedules on the following pages will help you prepare for your marathon. Choose the schedule that best reflects your targeted finish time. There are two schedules for each time goal: the first one presents the training distances in miles; the second in kilometres. A simple bar graph at the bottom of each page summarizes weekly changes in the distance of the long (Sunday) run and in the total weekly distance.

A word of caution is needed here: keep following your chosen program right up to the end. In too many cases, runners excited by the benefits of the early strength-building phase have pushed themselves too hard in the second half, only to end up on the injury list. Patience pays off—go easy, follow the program and the long-term rewards will be yours.

# To complete a marathon
## training program

### *kilometres*

| | SUN | MON | TUES | WED | THURS | FRI | SAT |
|---|---|---|---|---|---|---|---|
| **Week 1** | **10 km** long, slow run run 10 min/ walk 1 min | off | **6 km** tempo run 6:30 pace | **10 km** tempo run 85% effort | **6 km** steady run 6:50–7:10 pace | off | **6 km** steady easy run |
| **Week 2** | **10 km** long, slow run run 10 min/ walk 1 min | off | **6 km** tempo run 6:30 pace | **10 km** tempo run 85% effort | **6 km** steady run 6:50–7:10 pace | off | **6 km** steady easy run |
| **Week 3** | **13 km** long, slow run run 10 min/ walk 1 min | off | **6 km** tempo run 6:30 pace | **10 km** tempo run 85% effort | **8 km** steady run 6:50–7:10 pace | off | **6 km** steady easy run |
| **Week 4** | **13 km** long, slow run run 10 min/ walk 1 min | off | **6 km** tempo run 6:30 pace | **10 km** tempo run 85% effort | **8 km** steady run 6:50–7:10 pace | off | **6 km** steady easy run |
| **Week 5** | **16 km** long, slow run run 10 min/ walk 1 min | off | **6 km** tempo run 6:30 pace | **10 km** tempo run 85% effort | **8 km** steady run 6:50–7:10 pace | off | **6 km** steady easy run |
| **Week 6** | **16 km** long, slow run run 10 min/ walk 1 min | off | **6 km** tempo run 6:30 pace | **10 km** tempo run 85% effort | **8 km** steady run 6:50–7:10 pace | off | **6 km** steady easy run |
| **Week 7** | **19 km** long, slow run run 10 min/ walk 1 min | off | **6 km** tempo run 6:30 pace | **4 hills** 85% effort 3 km warm-up 3 km cool-down | **8 km** steady run 6:50–7:10 pace | off | **6 km** steady easy run |
| **Week 8** | **23 km** long, slow run run 10 min/ walk 1 min | off | **6 km** tempo run 6:30 pace | **5 hills** 85% effort 3 km warm-up 3 km cool-down | **10 km** steady run 6:50–7:10 pace | off | **6 km** steady easy run |
| **Week 9** | **26 km** long, slow run run 10 min/ walk 1 min | off | **6 km** tempo run 6:30 pace | **6 hills** 85% effort 3 km warm-up 3 km cool-down | **10 km** steady run 6:50–7:10 pace | off | **6 km** steady easy run |

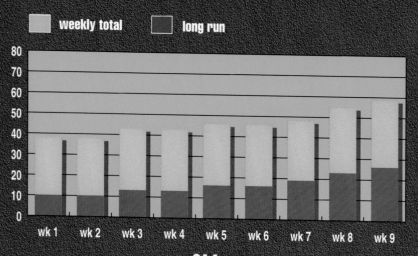

weekly total    long run

80
70
60
50
40
30
20
10
0

wk 1    wk 2    wk 3    wk 4    wk 5    wk 6    wk 7    wk 8    wk 9

**214**

# *kilometres*

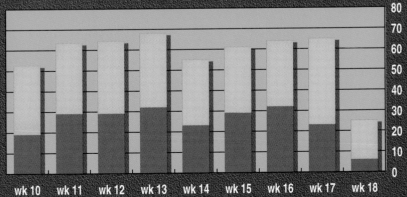

## To complete a marathon
*training program*

| | SUN | MON | TUES | WED | THURS | FRI | SAT |
|---|---|---|---|---|---|---|---|
| **Week 10** | **19 km** long, slow run run 10 min/ walk 1 min | off | **6 km** tempo run 6:30 pace | **7 hills** 85% effort 3 km warm-up 3 km cool-down | **10 km** steady run 6:50–7:10 pace | off | **6 km** steady easy run |
| **Week 11** | **29 km** long, slow run run 10 min/ walk 1 min | off | **6 km** tempo run 6:30 pace | **8 hills** 85% effort 3 km warm-up 3 km cool-down | **10 km** steady run 6:50–7:10 pace | off | **6 km** steady easy run |
| **Week 12** | **29 km** long, slow run run 10 min/ walk 1 min | off | **6 km** tempo run 6:30 pace | **9 hills** 85% effort 3 km warm-up 3 km cool-down | **10 km** steady run 6:50–7:10 pace | off | **6 km** steady easy run |
| **Week 13** | **32 km** long, slow run run 10 min/ walk 1 min | off | **6 km** tempo run 6:30 pace | **10 hills** 85% effort 3 km warm-up 3 km cool-down | **10 km** steady run 6:50–7:10 pace | off | **6 km** steady easy run |
| **Week 14** | **23 km** long, slow run run 10 min/ walk 1 min | off | **6 km** tempo run 6:30 pace | **10 km** fartlek 6:15–6:30 pace | **10 km** steady run 6:50–7:10 pace | off | **6 km** steady easy run |
| **Week 15** | **29 km** long, slow run run 10 min/ walk 1 min | off | **6 km** tempo run 6:30 pace | **10 km** fartlek 6:15–6:30 pace | **10 km** steady run 6:50–7:10 pace | off | **6 km** steady easy run |
| **Week 16** | **32 km** long, slow run run 10 min/ walk 1 min | off | **6 km** tempo run 6:30 pace | **10 km** fartlek 6:15–6:30 pace | **10 km** steady run 6:50–7:10 pace | off | **6 km** steady easy run |
| **Week 17** | **23 km** long, slow run run 10 min/ walk 1 min | off | **6 km** tempo run 6:30 pace | **10 km** fartlek 6:15–6:30 pace | **10 km** steady run 6:50–7:10 pace | off | **16 km** steady easy run |
| **Week 18** | **6 km** easy run run 10 min/ walk 1 min | off | **6 km** tempo run 6:30 pace | **10 km** steady run 6:30–7:10 pace | off | off | **3 km** steady easy run |
| **FINALE!** | **42 km** RACE DAY! | | | | | | |

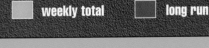

weekly total    long run

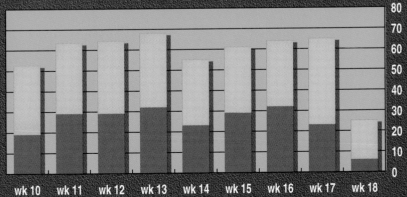

80
70
60
50
40
30
20
10
0

wk 10   wk 11   wk 12   wk 13   wk 14   wk 15   wk 16   wk 17   wk 18

215

# To complete a marathon
*training program*

miles

| | SUN | MON | TUES | WED | THURS | FRI | SAT |
|---|---|---|---|---|---|---|---|
| **Week 1** | **6 miles** long, slow run run 10 min/ walk 1 min | off | **4 miles** tempo run 10:30 pace | **6 miles** tempo run 85% effort | **4 miles** steady run 11:00–11:30 pace | off | **4 miles** steady easy run |
| **Week 2** | **6 miles** long, slow run run 10 min/ walk 1 min | off | **4 miles** tempo run 10:30 pace | **6 miles** tempo run 85% effort | **4 miles** steady run 11:00–11:30 pace | off | **4 miles** steady easy run |
| **Week 3** | **8 miles** long, slow run run 10 min/ walk 1 min | off | **4 miles** tempo run 10:30 pace | **6 miles** tempo run 85% effort | **5 miles** steady run 11:00–11:30 pace | off | **4 miles** steady easy run |
| **Week 4** | **8 miles** long, slow run run 10 min/ walk 1 min | off | **4 miles** tempo run 10:30 pace | **6 miles** tempo run 85% effort | **5 miles** steady run 11:00–11:30 pace | off | **4 miles** steady easy run |
| **Week 5** | **10 miles** long, slow run run 10 min/ walk 1 min | off | **4 miles** tempo run 10:30 pace | **6 miles** tempo run 85% effort | **5 miles** steady run 11:00–11:30 pace | off | **4 miles** steady easy run |
| **Week 6** | **10 miles** long, slow run run 10 min/ walk 1 min | off | **4 miles** tempo run 10:30 pace | **6 miles** tempo run 85% effort | **5 miles** steady run 11:00–11:30 pace | off | **4 miles** steady easy run |
| **Week 7** | **12 miles** long, slow run run 10 min/ walk 1 min | off | **4 miles** tempo run 10:30 pace | **4 hills** 85% effort 2 mi warm-up 2 mi cool-down | **5 miles** steady run 11:00–11:30 pace | off | **4 miles** steady easy run |
| **Week 8** | **14 miles** long, slow run run 10 min/ walk 1 min | off | **4 miles** tempo run 10:30 pace | **5 hills** 85% effort 2 mi warm-up 2 mi cool-down | **6 miles** steady run 11:00–11:30 pace | off | **4 miles** steady easy run |
| **Week 9** | **16 miles** long, slow run run 10 min/ walk 1 min | off | **4 miles** tempo run 10:30 pace | **6 hills** 85% effort 2 mi warm-up 2 mi cool-down | **6 miles** steady run 11:00–11:30 pace | off | **4 miles** steady easy run |

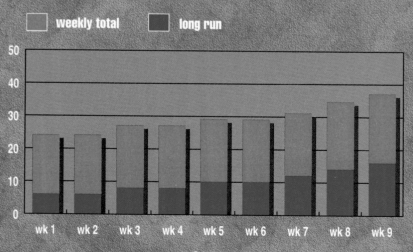

weekly total  long run

# miles

# To complete a marathon
*training program*

|  | SUN | MON | TUES | WED | THURS | FRI | SAT |
|---|---|---|---|---|---|---|---|
| **Week 10** | **12 miles** long, slow run run 10 min/ walk 1 min | off | **4 miles** tempo run 10:30 pace | **7 hills** 85% effort 2 mi warm-up 2 mi cool-down | **6 miles** steady run 11:00–11:30 pace | off | **4 miles** steady easy run |
| **Week 11** | **18 miles** long, slow run run 10 min/ walk 1 min | off | **4 miles** tempo run 10:30 pace | **8 hills** 85% effort 2 mi warm-up 2 mi cool-down | **6 miles** steady run 11:00–11:30 pace | off | **4 miles** steady easy run |
| **Week 12** | **18 miles** long, slow run run 10 min/ walk 1 min | off | **4 miles** tempo run 10:30 pace | **9 hills** 85% effort 2 mi warm-up 2 mi cool-down | **6 miles** steady run 11:00–11:30 pace | off | **4 miles** steady easy run |
| **Week 13** | **20 miles** long, slow run run 10 min/ walk 1 min | off | **4 miles** tempo run 10:30 pace | **10 hills** 85% effort 2 mi warm-up 2 mi cool-down | **6 miles** steady run 11:00–11:30 pace | off | **4 miles** steady easy run |
| **Week 14** | **14 miles** long, slow run run 10 min/ walk 1 min | off | **4 miles** tempo run 10:30 pace | **6 miles** fartlek 10:00–11:00 pace | **6 miles** steady run 11:00–11:30 pace | off | **4 miles** steady easy run |
| **Week 15** | **18 miles** long, slow run run 10 min/ walk 1 min | off | **4 miles** tempo run 10:30 pace | **6 miles** fartlek 10:00–11:00 pace | **6 miles** steady run 11:00–11:30 pace | off | **4 miles** steady easy run |
| **Week 16** | **20 miles** long, slow run run 10 min/ walk 1 min | off | **4 miles** tempo run 10:30 pace | **6 miles** fartlek 10:00–11:00 pace | **6 miles** steady run 11:00–11:30 pace | off | **4 miles** steady easy run |
| **Week 17** | **14 miles** long, slow run run 10 min/ walk 1 min | off | **4 miles** tempo run 10:30 pace | **6 miles** fartlek 10:00–11:00 pace | **6 miles** steady run 11:00–11:30 pace | off | **10 miles** tempo run 10:30–11:30 pace |
| **Week 18** | **4 miles** easy run run 10 min/ walk 1 min | off | **4 miles** tempo run 10:30 pace | **6 miles** tempo run 10:30 pace | off | off | **2 miles** steady easy run |
| **FINALE!** | **26 miles** RACE DAY! | | | | | | |

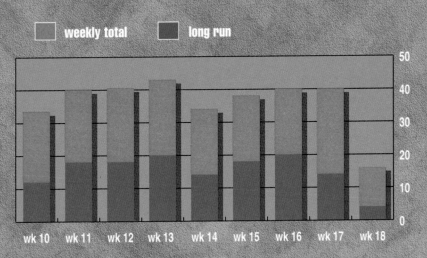

■ weekly total     ■ long run

# 4 hr. 30 min. marathon

*training program*

**kilometres**

| | SUN | MON | TUES | WED | THURS | FRI | SAT |
|---|---|---|---|---|---|---|---|
| **Week 1** | **10 km**<br>long, slow run<br>run 10 min/<br>walk 1 min | off | **6 km**<br>tempo run<br>6:20 pace | **10 km**<br>tempo run<br>85% effort | **6 km**<br>steady run<br>6:30–7:10 pace | off | **6 km**<br>steady<br>easy run |
| **Week 2** | **10 km**<br>long, slow run<br>run 10 min/<br>walk 1 min | off | **6 km**<br>tempo run<br>6:20 pace | **10 km**<br>tempo run<br>85% effort | **6 km**<br>steady run<br>6:30–7:10 pace | off | **6 km**<br>steady<br>easy run |
| **Week 3** | **13 km**<br>long, slow run<br>run 10 min/<br>walk 1 min | off | **6 km**<br>tempo run<br>6:20 pace | **10 km**<br>tempo run<br>85% effort | **8 km**<br>steady run<br>6:30-7:10 pace | off | **6 km**<br>steady<br>easy run |
| **Week 4** | **13 km**<br>long, slow run<br>run 10 min/<br>walk 1 min | off | **6 km**<br>tempo run<br>6:20 pace | **10 km**<br>tempo run<br>85% effort | **8 km**<br>steady run<br>6:30–7:10 pace | off | **6 km**<br>steady<br>easy run |
| **Week 5** | **16 km**<br>long, slow run<br>run 10 min/<br>walk 1 min | off | **6 km**<br>tempo run<br>6:20 pace | **10 km**<br>tempo run<br>85% effort | **8 km**<br>steady run<br>6:30–7:10 pace | off | **6 km**<br>steady<br>easy run |
| **Week 6** | **16 km**<br>long, slow run<br>run 10 min/<br>walk 1 min | off | **6 km**<br>tempo run<br>6:20 pace | **10 km**<br>tempo run<br>85% effort | **8 km**<br>steady run<br>6:30–7:10 pace | off | **6 km**<br>steady<br>easy run |
| **Week 7** | **19 km**<br>long, slow run<br>run 10 min/<br>walk 1 min | off | **6 km**<br>tempo run<br>6:20 pace | **4 hills**<br>85% effort<br>3 km warm-up<br>3 km cool-down | **8 km**<br>steady run<br>6:30–7:10 pace | off | **6 km**<br>steady<br>easy run |
| **Week 8** | **23 km**<br>long, slow run<br>run 10 min/<br>walk 1 min | off | **6 km**<br>tempo run<br>6:20 pace | **5 hills**<br>85% effort<br>3 km warm-up<br>3 km cool-down | **8 km**<br>steady run<br>6:30–7:10 pace | off | **6 km**<br>steady<br>easy run |
| **Week 9** | **26 km**<br>long, slow run<br>run 10 min/<br>walk 1 min | off | **6 km**<br>tempo run<br>6:20 pace | **6 hills**<br>85% effort<br>3 km warm-up<br>3 km cool-down | **8 km**<br>steady run<br>6:30–7:10 pace | off | **6 km**<br>steady<br>easy run |

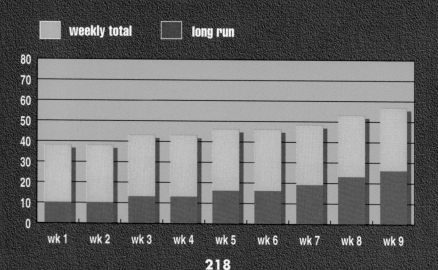

□ weekly total   ■ long run

# *kilometres*    4 hr. 30 min. marathon
### *training program*

|  | SUN | MON | TUES | WED | THURS | FRI | SAT |
|---|---|---|---|---|---|---|---|
| **Week 10** | **19 km** long, slow run run 10 min/ walk 1 min | off | **6 km** tempo run 6:20 pace | **7 hills** 85% effort 3 km warm-up 3 km cool-down | **8 km** steady run 6:30–7:10 pace | off | **6 km** steady easy run |
| **Week 11** | **29 km** long, slow run run 10 min/ walk 1 min | off | **6 km** tempo run 6:20 pace | **8 hills** 85% effort 3 km warm-up 3 km cool-down | **8 km** steady run 6:30–7:10 pace | off | **6 km** steady easy run |
| **Week 12** | **29 km** long, slow run run 10 min/ walk 1 min | off | **6 km** tempo run 6:20 pace | **9 hills** 85% effort 3 km warm-up 3 km cool-down | **8 km** steady run 6:30–7:10 pace | off | **6 km** steady easy run |
| **Week 13** | **32 km** long, slow run run 10 min/ walk 1 min | off | **6 km** tempo run 6:20 pace | **10 hills** 85% effort 3 km warm-up 3 km cool-down | **8 km** steady run 6:30–7:10 pace | off | **6 km** steady easy run |
| **Week 14** | **23 km** long, slow run run 10 min/ walk 1 min | off | **6 km** tempo run 6:20 pace | **10 km** fartlek 6:00–6:15 pace | **8 km** steady run 6:30–7:10 pace | off | **6 km** steady easy run |
| **Week 15** | **29 km** long, slow run run 10 min/ walk 1 min | off | **6 km** tempo run 6:20 pace | **10 km** fartlek 6:00–6:15 pace | **10 km** steady run 6:30–7:10 pace | off | **6 km** steady easy run |
| **Week 16** | **32 km** long, slow run run 10 min/ walk 1 min | off | **6 km** tempo run 6:20 pace | **10 km** fartlek 6:00–6:15 pace | **10 km** steady run 6:30–7:10 pace | off | **6 km** steady easy run |
| **Week 17** | **23 km** long, slow run run 10 min/ walk 1 min | off | **6 km** tempo run 6:20 pace | **10 km** fartlek 6:00–6:15 pace | **10 km** steady run 6:30–7:10 pace | off | **16 km** run/walk race pace (6:20 pace) |
| **Week 18** | **6 km** easy run | off | **6 km** race pace (6:20 pace) | **10 km** race pace (6:20 pace) | off | off | **3 km** steady easy run |
| **FINALE!** | **42 km** RACE DAY! 6:24 pace |  |  |  |  |  |  |

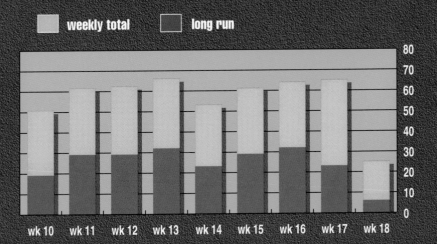

weekly total    long run

wk 10   wk 11   wk 12   wk 13   wk 14   wk 15   wk 16   wk 17   wk 18

# 4 hr. 30 min. marathon
## training program

*miles*

| | SUN | MON | TUES | WED | THURS | FRI | SAT |
|---|---|---|---|---|---|---|---|
| **Week 1** | **6 miles** long, slow run run 10 min/ walk 1 min | off | **4 miles** tempo run 10:00 pace | **6 miles** tempo run 85% effort | **4 miles** steady run 10:30–11:30 pace | off | **4 miles** steady easy run |
| **Week 2** | **6 miles** long, slow run run 10 min/ walk 1 min | off | **4 miles** tempo run 10:00 pace | **6 miles** tempo run 85% effort | **4 miles** steady run 10:30–11:30 pace | off | **4 miles** steady easy run |
| **Week 3** | **8 miles** long, slow run run 10 min/ walk 1 min | off | **4 miles** tempo run 10:00 pace | **6 miles** tempo run 85% effort | **5 miles** steady run 10:30–11:30 pace | off | **4 miles** steady easy run |
| **Week 4** | **8 miles** long, slow run run 10 min/ walk 1 min | off | **4 miles** tempo run 10:00 pace | **6 miles** tempo run 85% effort | **5 miles** steady run 10:30–11:30 pace | off | **4 miles** steady easy run |
| **Week 5** | **10 miles** long, slow run run 10 min/ walk 1 min | off | **4 miles** tempo run 10:00 pace | **6 miles** tempo run 85% effort | **5 miles** steady run 10:30–11:30 pace | off | **4 miles** steady easy run |
| **Week 6** | **10 miles** long, slow run run 10 min/ walk 1 min | off | **4 miles** tempo run 10:00 pace | **6 miles** tempo run 85% effort | **5 miles** steady run 10:30–11:30 pace | off | **4 miles** steady easy run |
| **Week 7** | **12 miles** long, slow run run 10 min/ walk 1 min | off | **4 miles** tempo run 10:00 pace | **4 hills** 85% effort 2 mi warm-up 2 mi cool-down | **5 miles** steady run 10:30–11:30 pace | off | **4 miles** steady easy run |
| **Week 8** | **14 miles** long, slow run run 10 min/ walk 1 min | off | **4 miles** tempo run 10:00 pace | **5 hills** 85% effort 2 mi warm-up 2 mi cool-down | **5 miles** steady run 10:30–11:30 pace | off | **4 miles** steady easy run |
| **Week 9** | **16 miles** long, slow run run 10 min/ walk 1 min | off | **4 miles** tempo run 10:00 pace | **6 hills** 85% effort 2 mi warm-up 2 mi cool-down | **5 miles** steady run 10:30–11:30 pace | off | **4 miles** steady easy run |

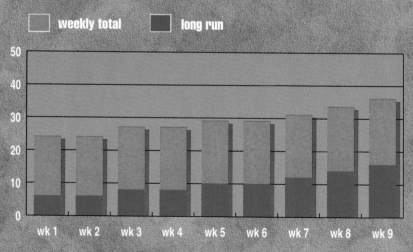

□ weekly total  ■ long run

# 4 hr. 30 min. marathon
*training program*

| | SUN | MON | TUES | WED | THURS | FRI | SAT |
|---|---|---|---|---|---|---|---|
| **Week 10** | **12 miles** long, slow run run 10 min/ walk 1 min | off | **4 miles** tempo run 10:00 pace | **7 hills** 85% effort 2 mi warm-up 2 mi cool-down | **5 miles** steady run 10:30–11:30 pace | off | **4 miles** steady easy run |
| **Week 11** | **18 miles** long, slow run run 10 min/ walk 1 min | off | **4 miles** tempo run 10:00 pace | **8 hills** 85% effort 2 mi warm-up 2 mi cool-down | **5 miles** steady run 10:30–11:30 pace | off | **4 miles** steady easy run |
| **Week 12** | **18 miles** long, slow run run 10 min/ walk 1 min | off | **4 miles** tempo run 10:00 pace | **9 hills** 85% effort 2 mi warm-up 2 mi cool-down | **5 miles** steady run 10:30–11:30 pace | off | **4 miles** steady easy run |
| **Week 13** | **20 miles** long, slow run run 10 min/ walk 1 min | off | **4 miles** tempo run 10:00 pace | **10 hills** 85% effort 2 mi warm-up 2 mi cool-down | **5 miles** steady run 10:30–11:30 pace | off | **4 miles** steady easy run |
| **Week 14** | **14 miles** long, slow run run 10 min/ walk 1 min | off | **4 miles** tempo run 10:00 pace | **6 miles** fartlek 9:30–10:30 pace | **5 miles** steady run 10:30–11:30 pace | off | **4 miles** steady easy run |
| **Week 15** | **18 miles** long, slow run run 10 min/ walk 1 min | off | **4 miles** tempo run 10:00 pace | **6 miles** fartlek 9:30–10:30 pace | **6 miles** steady run 10:30–11:30 pace | off | **4 miles** steady easy run |
| **Week 16** | **20 miles** long, slow run run 10 min/ walk 1 min | off | **4 miles** tempo run 10:00 pace | **6 miles** fartlek 9:30–10:30 pace | **6 miles** steady run 10:30–11:30 pace | off | **4 miles** steady easy run |
| **Week 17** | **14 miles** long, slow run run 10 min/ walk 1 min | off | **4 miles** tempo run 10:00 pace | **6 miles** fartlek 9:30–10:30 pace | **6 miles** steady run 10:30–11:30 pace | off | **10 miles** run/walk race pace (10:20 pace) |
| **Week 18** | **4 miles** easy run | off | **4 miles** race pace (10:20 pace) | **6 miles** race pace (10:20 pace) | off | off | **2 miles** steady easy run |
| **FINALE!** | **26 miles** RACE DAY! 10:18 pace | | | | | | |

**weekly total**  **long run**

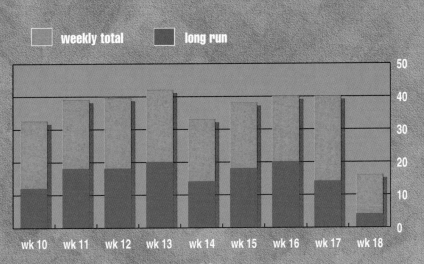

| wk 10 | wk 11 | wk 12 | wk 13 | wk 14 | wk 15 | wk 16 | wk 17 | wk 18 |

# 4 hr. marathon
*training program*

*kilometres*

| | SUN | MON | TUES | WED | THURS | FRI | SAT |
|---|---|---|---|---|---|---|---|
| **Week 1** | **10 km** run 10 min/ walk 1 min 6:30 pace | off | **6 km** tempo run 5:50 pace | **10 km** tempo run 85% effort | **6 km** steady run 5:55 pace | off | **6 km** steady easy run |
| **Week 2** | **10 km** run 10 min/ walk 1 min 6:30 pace | off | **6 km** tempo run 5:50 pace | **10 km** tempo run 85% effort | **6 km** steady run 5:55 pace | off | **6 km** steady easy run |
| **Week 3** | **13 km** run 10 min/ walk 1 min 6:30 pace | off | **6 km** tempo run 5:50 pace | **10 km** tempo run 85% effort | **8 km** steady run 5:55 pace | off | **6 km** steady easy run |
| **Week 4** | **13 km** run 10 min/ walk 1 min 6:30 pace | off | **6 km** tempo run 5:50 pace | **10 km** tempo run 85% effort | **8 km** steady run 5:55 pace | off | **6 km** steady easy run |
| **Week 5** | **16 km** run 10 min/ walk 1 min 6:30 pace | off | **6 km** tempo run 5:50 pace | **10 km** tempo run 85% effort | **8 km** steady run 5:55 pace | off | **6 km** steady easy run |
| **Week 6** | **16 km** run 10 min/ walk 1 min 6:30 pace | off | **6 km** tempo run 5:50 pace | **10 km** tempo run 85% effort | **8 km** steady run 5:55 pace | off | **6 km** steady easy run |
| **Week 7** | **19 km** run 10 min/ walk 1 min 6:30 pace | off | **6 km** tempo run 5:50 pace | **4 hills** 85% effort 3 km warm-up 3 km cool-down | **8 km** steady run 5:55 pace | off | **6 km** steady easy run |
| **Week 8** | **23 km** run 10 min/ walk 1 min 6:30 pace | off | **6 km** tempo run 5:50 pace | **5 hills** 85% effort 3 km warm-up 3 km cool-down | **8 km** steady run 5:55 pace | off | **6 km** steady easy run |
| **Week 9** | **26 km** run 10 min/ walk 1 min 6:30 pace | off | **6 km** tempo run 5:50 pace | **6 hills** 85% effort 3 km warm-up 3 km cool-down | **10 km** steady run 5:55 pace | off | **6 km** steady easy run |

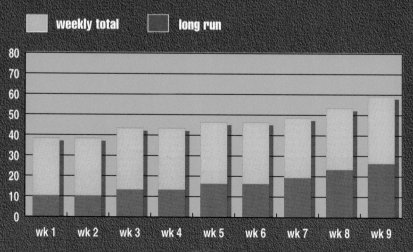

weekly total ▫ long run

80
70
60
50
40
30
20
10
0

wk 1   wk 2   wk 3   wk 4   wk 5   wk 6   wk 7   wk 8   wk 9

## kilometres

# 4 hr. marathon
*training program*

| | SUN | MON | TUES | WED | THURS | FRI | SAT |
|---|---|---|---|---|---|---|---|
| **Week 10** | **19 km** run 10 min/ walk 1 min 6:30 pace | off | **6 km** tempo run 5:50 pace | **7 hills** 85% effort 3 km warm-up 3 km cool-down | **10 km** steady run 5:55 pace | off | **6 km** steady easy run |
| **Week 11** | **29 km** run 10 min/ walk 1 min 6:30 pace | off | **6 km** tempo run 5:50 pace | **8 hills** 85% effort 3 km warm-up 3 km cool-down | **10 km** steady run 5:55 pace | off | **6 km** steady easy run |
| **Week 12** | **29 km** run 10 min/ walk 1 min 6:30 pace | off | **6 km** tempo run 5:50 pace | **9 hills** 85% effort 3 km warm-up 3 km cool-down | **10 km** steady run 5:55 pace | off | **6 km** steady easy run |
| **Week 13** | **32 km** run 10 min/ walk 1 min 6:30 pace | off | **6 km** tempo run 5:50 pace | **10 hills** 85% effort 3 km warm-up 3 km cool-down | **10 km** steady run 5:55 pace | off | **6 km** steady easy run |
| **Week 14** | **23 km** run 10 min/ walk 1 min 6:30 pace | off | **6 km** tempo run 5:50 pace | **10 km** fartlek 5:15–5:55 pace | **10 km** steady run 5:55 pace | off | **6 km** steady easy run |
| **Week 15** | **29 km** run 10 min/ walk 1 min 6:30 pace | off | **6 km** tempo run 5:50 pace | **10 km** fartlek 5:15–5:55 pace | **10 km** steady run 5:55 pace | off | **6 km** steady easy run |
| **Week 16** | **32 km** run 10 min/ walk 1 min 6:30 pace | off | **6 km** tempo run 5:50 pace | **10 km** fartlek 5:15–5:55 pace | **10 km** steady run 5:55 pace | off | **6 km** steady easy run |
| **Week 17** | **23 km** run 10 min/ walk 1 min 6:30 pace | off | **6 km** tempo run 5:50 pace | **10 km** fartlek 5:15–5:55 pace | **10 km** steady run 5:55 pace | off | **16 km** run/walk race pace (5:40 pace) |
| **Week 18** | **6 km** easy run 6:30 pace | off | **6 km** race pace (5:40 pace) | **10 km** race pace (5:40 pace) | off | off | **3 km** steady easy run |
| **FINALE!** | **42 km** RACE DAY! 5:41 pace | | | | | | |

weekly total · long run

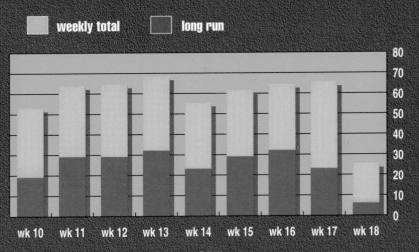

wk 10 · wk 11 · wk 12 · wk 13 · wk 14 · wk 15 · wk 16 · wk 17 · wk 18

**223**

# 4 hr. marathon
*training program*

*miles*

| | SUN | MON | TUES | WED | THURS | FRI | SAT |
|---|---|---|---|---|---|---|---|
| **Week 1** | **6 miles** run 10 min/ walk 1 min 10:30 pace | off | **4 miles** tempo run 9:20 pace | **6 miles** tempo run 85% effort | **4 miles** steady run 9:30 pace | off | **4 miles** steady easy run |
| **Week 2** | **6 miles** run 10 min/ walk 1 min 10:30 pace | off | **4 miles** tempo run 9:20 pace | **6 miles** tempo run 85% effort | **4 miles** steady run 9:30 pace | off | **4 miles** steady easy run |
| **Week 3** | **8 miles** run 10 min/ walk 1 min 10:30 pace | off | **4 miles** tempo run 9:20 pace | **6 miles** tempo run 85% effort | **5 miles** steady run 9:30 pace | off | **4 miles** steady easy run |
| **Week 4** | **8 miles** run 10 min/ walk 1 min 10:30 pace | off | **4 miles** tempo run 9:20 pace | **6 miles** tempo run 85% effort | **5 miles** steady run 9:30 pace | off | **4 miles** steady easy run |
| **Week 5** | **10 miles** run 10 min/ walk 1 min 10:30 pace | off | **4 miles** tempo run 9:20 pace | **6 miles** tempo run 85% effort | **5 miles** steady run 9:30 pace | off | **4 miles** steady easy run |
| **Week 6** | **10 miles** run 10 min/ walk 1 min 10:30 pace | off | **4 miles** tempo run 9:20 pace | **6 miles** tempo run 85% effort | **5 miles** steady run 9:30 pace | off | **4 miles** steady easy run |
| **Week 7** | **12 miles** run 10 min/ walk 1 min 10:30 pace | off | **4 miles** tempo run 9:20 pace | **4 hills** 85% effort 2 mi warm-up 2 mi cool-down | **5 miles** steady run 9:30 pace | off | **4 miles** steady easy run |
| **Week 8** | **14 miles** run 10 min/ walk 1 min 10:30 pace | off | **4 miles** tempo run 9:20 pace | **5 hills** 85% effort 2 mi warm-up 2 mi cool-down | **5 miles** steady run 9:30 pace | off | **4 miles** steady easy run |
| **Week 9** | **16 miles** run 10 min/ walk 1 min 10:30 pace | off | **4 miles** tempo run 9:20 pace | **6 hills** 85% effort 2 mi warm-up 2 mi cool-down | **6 miles** steady run 9:30 pace | off | **4 miles** steady easy run |

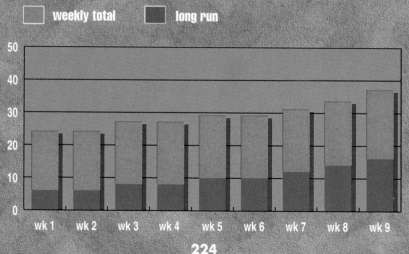

weekly total        long run

# 4 hr. marathon
*training program*

| | SUN | MON | TUES | WED | THURS | FRI | SAT |
|---|---|---|---|---|---|---|---|
| **Week 10** | **12 miles** run 10 min/ walk 1 min 10:30 pace | off | **4 miles** tempo run 9:20 pace | **7 hills** 85% effort 2 mi warm-up 2 mi cool-down | **6 miles** steady run 9:30 pace | off | **4 miles** steady easy run |
| **Week 11** | **18 miles** run 10 min/ walk 1 min 10:30 pace | off | **4 miles** tempo run 9:20 pace | **8 hills** 85% effort 2 mi warm-up 2 mi cool-down | **6 miles** steady run 9:30 pace | off | **4 miles** steady easy run |
| **Week 12** | **18 miles** run 10 min/ walk 1 min 10:30 pace | off | **4 miles** tempo run 9:20 pace | **9 hills** 85% effort 2 mi warm-up 2 mi cool-down | **6 miles** steady run 9:30 pace | off | **4 miles** steady easy run |
| **Week 13** | **20 miles** run 10 min/ walk 1 min 10:30 pace | off | **4 miles** tempo run 9:20 pace | **10 hills** 85% effort 2 mi warm-up 2 mi cool-down | **6 miles** steady run 9:30 pace | off | **4 miles** steady easy run |
| **Week 14** | **14 miles** run 10 min/ walk 1 min 10:30 pace | off | **4 miles** tempo run 9:20 pace | **6 miles** fartlek 8:30–9:30 pace | **6 miles** steady run 9:30 pace | off | **4 miles** steady easy run |
| **Week 15** | **18 miles** run 10 min/ walk 1 min 10:30 pace | off | **4 miles** tempo run 9:20 pace | **6 miles** fartlek 8:30–9:30 pace | **6 miles** steady run 9:30 pace | off | **4 miles** steady easy run |
| **Week 16** | **20 miles** run 10 min/ walk 1 min 10:30 pace | off | **4 miles** tempo run 9:20 pace | **6 miles** fartlek 8:30–9:30 pace | **6 miles** steady run 9:30 pace | off | **4 miles** steady easy run |
| **Week 17** | **14 miles** run 10 min/ walk 1 min 10:30 pace | off | **4 miles** tempo run 9:20 pace | *am* **6 miles** fartlek 8:30–9:30 pace | **6 miles** steady run 9:30 pace | off | **10 miles** run/walk race pace (9:05 pace) |
| **Week 18** | **4 miles** easy run 10:30 pace | off | **4 miles** race pace (9:05 pace) | **6 miles** race pace (9:05 pace) | off | off | **2 miles** steady easy run |
| **FINALE!** | **26 miles** RACE DAY! 9:09 pace | | | | | | |

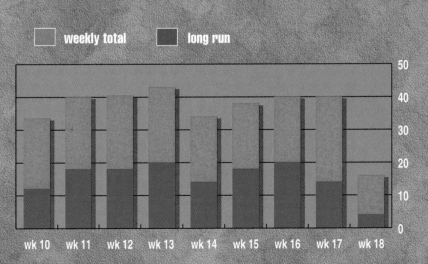

☐ **weekly total**   ■ **long run**

# 3 hr. 45 min. marathon
*training program*

*kilometres*

| | SUN | MON | TUES | WED | THURS | FRI | SAT |
|---|---|---|---|---|---|---|---|
| Week 1 | 10 km<br>run 10 min/<br>walk 1 min<br>5:45–6:30 pace | off | 6 km<br>tempo run<br>5:25 pace | 10 km<br>tempo run<br>85% effort | 8 km<br>steady run<br>5:35 pace | 10 km<br>fartlek<br>5:05–5:30 pace | 6 km<br>steady<br>easy run |
| Week 2 | 13 km<br>run 10 min/<br>walk 1 min<br>5:45–6:30 pace | off | 6 km<br>tempo run<br>5:25 pace | 10 km<br>tempo run<br>85% effort | 8 km<br>steady run<br>5:35 pace | 10 km<br>fartlek<br>5:05–5:30 pace | 6 km<br>steady<br>easy run |
| Week 3 | 13 km<br>run 10 min/<br>walk 1 min<br>5:45–6:30 pace | off | 6 km<br>tempo run<br>5:25 pace | 10 km<br>tempo run<br>85% effort | 8 km<br>steady run<br>5:35 pace | 10 km<br>fartlek<br>5:05–5:30 pace | 6 km<br>steady<br>easy run |
| Week 4 | 13 km<br>run 10 min/<br>walk 1 min<br>5:45–6:30 pace | off | 6 km<br>tempo run<br>5:25 pace | 10 km<br>tempo run<br>85% effort | 8 km<br>steady run<br>5:35 pace | 10 km<br>fartlek<br>5:05–5:30 pace | 6 km<br>steady<br>easy run |
| Week 5 | 16 km<br>run 10 min/<br>walk 1 min<br>5:45–6:30 pace | off | 6 km<br>tempo run<br>5:25 pace | 10 km<br>tempo run<br>85% effort | 8 km<br>steady run<br>5:35 pace | 10 km<br>fartlek<br>5:05–5:30 pace | 6 km<br>steady<br>easy run |
| Week 6 | 16 km<br>run 10 min/<br>walk 1 min<br>5:45–6:30 pace | off | 6 km<br>tempo run<br>5:25 pace | 10 km<br>tempo run<br>85% effort | 8 km<br>steady run<br>5:35 pace | 10 km<br>fartlek<br>5:05–5:30 pace | 6 km<br>steady<br>easy run |
| Week 7 | 19 km<br>run 10 min/<br>walk 1 min<br>5:45–6:30 pace | off | 6 km<br>tempo run<br>5:25 pace | 4 hills<br>85% effort<br>3 km warm-up<br>3 km cool-down | 8 km<br>steady run<br>5:35 pace | 10 km<br>fartlek<br>5:05–5:30 pace | 6 km<br>steady<br>easy run |
| Week 8 | 23 km<br>run 10 min/<br>walk 1 min<br>5:45–6:30 pace | off | 10 km<br>tempo run<br>5:25 pace | 5 hills<br>85% effort<br>3 km warm-up<br>3 km cool-down | 6 km<br>steady run<br>5:35 pace | 10 km<br>fartlek<br>5:05–5:30 pace | 6 km<br>steady<br>easy run |
| Week 9 | 22 km<br>run 10 min/<br>walk 1 min<br>5:45–6:30 pace | off | 10 km<br>tempo run<br>5:25 pace | 6 hills<br>85% effort<br>3 km warm-up<br>3 km cool-down | 6 km<br>steady run<br>5:35 pace | 10 km<br>fartlek<br>5:05–5:30 pace | 6 km<br>steady<br>easy run |

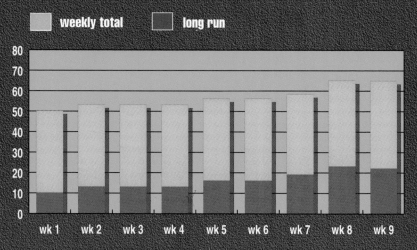

weekly total    long run

wk 1   wk 2   wk 3   wk 4   wk 5   wk 6   wk 7   wk 8   wk 9

| | SUN | MON | TUES | WED | THURS | FRI | SAT |
|---|---|---|---|---|---|---|---|
| **Week 10** | **19 km** run 10 min/ walk 1 min 5:45–6:30 pace | off | **10 km** tempo run 5:25 pace | **7 hills** 85% effort 3 km warm-up 3 km cool-down | **6 km** steady run 5:35 pace | **10 km** fartlek 5:05–5:30 pace | **6 km** steady easy run |
| **Week 11** | **26 km** run 10 min/ walk 1 min 5:45–6:30 pace | off | **6 km** tempo run 5:25 pace | **8 hills** 85% effort 3 km warm-up 3 km cool-down | **8 km** steady run 5:35 pace | **10 km** fartlek 5:05–5:30 pace | **6 km** steady easy run |
| **Week 12** | **29 km** run 10 min/ walk 1 min 5:45–6:30 pace | off | **6 km** tempo run 5:25 pace | **9 hills** 85% effort 3 km warm-up 3 km cool-down | **6 km** steady run 5:35 pace | **10 km** fartlek 5:05–5:30 pace | **6 km** steady easy run |
| **Week 13** | **32 km** run 10 min/ walk 1 min 5:45–6:30 pace | off | **6 km** tempo run 5:25 pace | **10 hills** 85% effort 3 km warm-up 3 km cool-down | **6 km** steady run 5:35 pace | **10 km** fartlek 5:05–5:30 pace | **6 km** steady easy run |
| **Week 14** | **23 km** run 10 min/ walk 1 min 5:45–6:30 pace | off | **6 km** tempo run 5:25 pace | **2 speed int.** 1.6 km @ 4:35/km 3 km warm-up 3 km cool-down | **8 km** steady run 5:35 pace | **10 km** fartlek 5:05–5:30 pace | **6 km** steady easy run |
| **Week 15** | **29 km** run 10 min/ walk 1 min 5:45–6:30 pace | off | **6 km** tempo run 5:25 pace | **3 speed int.** 1.6 km @ 4:35/km 3 km warm-up 3 km cool-down | **6 km** steady run 5:35 pace | **10 km** fartlek 5:05–5:30 pace | **6 km** steady easy run |
| **Week 16** | **32 km** run 10 min/ walk 1 min 5:45–6:30 pace | off | **6 km** tempo run 5:25 pace | **4 speed int.** 1.6 km @ 4:35/km 3 km warm-up 3 km cool-down | **6 km** steady run 5:35 pace | **10 km** fartlek 5:05–5:30 pace | **6 km** steady easy run |
| **Week 17** | **23 km** run 10 min/ walk 1 min 5:45–6:30 pace | off | **6 km** tempo run 5:25 pace | **5 speed int.** 1.6 km @ 4:35/km 3 km warm-up 3 km cool-down | **6 km** steady run 5:35 pace | **10 km** fartlek 5:05–5:30 pace | **16 km** race pace (5:20 pace) |
| **Week 18** | **6 km** easy run 5:45–6:30 pace | off | **6 km** race pace (5:20 pace) | **10 km** race pace (5:20 pace) | off | off | **3 km** steady easy run |
| **FINALE!** | **42 km** RACE DAY! 5:20 pace | | | | | | |

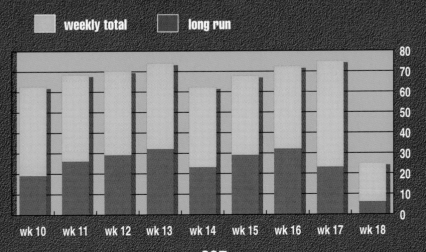

weekly total     long run

# 3 hr. 45 min. marathon
## training program

*miles*

| | SUN | MON | TUES | WED | THURS | FRI | SAT |
|---|---|---|---|---|---|---|---|
| **Week 1** | 6 miles<br>run 10 min/<br>walk 1 min<br>9:15–10:30 pace | off | 4 miles<br>tempo run<br>8:45 pace | 6 miles<br>tempo run<br>85% effort | 4 miles<br>steady run<br>9:00 pace | 6 miles<br>fartlek<br>8:15–8:45 pace | 4 miles<br>steady<br>easy run |
| **Week 2** | 8 miles<br>run 10 min/<br>walk 1 min<br>9:15–10:30 pace | off | 4 miles<br>tempo run<br>8:45 pace | 6 miles<br>tempo run<br>85% effort | 4 miles<br>steady run<br>9:00 pace | 6 miles<br>fartlek<br>8:15–8:45 pace | 4 miles<br>steady<br>easy run |
| **Week 3** | 8 miles<br>run 10 min/<br>walk 1 min<br>9:15–10:30 pace | off | 4 miles<br>tempo run<br>8:45 pace | 6 miles<br>tempo run<br>85% effort | 5 miles<br>steady run<br>9:00 pace | 6 miles<br>fartlek<br>8:15–8:45 pace | 4 miles<br>steady<br>easy run |
| **Week 4** | 8 miles<br>run 10 min/<br>walk 1 min<br>9:15–10:30 pace | off | 4 miles<br>tempo run<br>8:45 pace | 6 miles<br>tempo run<br>85% effort | 5 miles<br>steady run<br>9:00 pace | 6 miles<br>fartlek<br>8:15–8:45 pace | 4 miles<br>steady<br>easy run |
| **Week 5** | 10 miles<br>run 10 min/<br>walk 1 min<br>9:15–10:30 pace | off | 4 miles<br>tempo run<br>8:45 pace | 6 miles<br>tempo run<br>85% effort | 5 miles<br>steady run<br>9:00 pace | 6 miles<br>fartlek<br>8:15–8:45 pace | 4 miles<br>steady<br>easy run |
| **Week 6** | 10 miles<br>run 10 min/<br>walk 1 min<br>9:15–10:30 pace | off | 4 miles<br>tempo run<br>8:45 pace | 6 miles<br>tempo run<br>85% effort | 5 miles<br>steady run<br>9:00 pace | 6 miles<br>fartlek<br>8:15–8:45 pace | 4 miles<br>steady<br>easy run |
| **Week 7** | 12 miles<br>run 10 min/<br>walk 1 min<br>9:15–10:30 pace | off | 4 miles<br>tempo run<br>8:45 pace | 4 hills<br>85% effort<br>2 mi warm-up<br>2 mi cool-down | 5 miles<br>steady run<br>9:00 pace | 6 miles<br>fartlek<br>8:15–8:45 pace | 4 miles<br>steady<br>easy run |
| **Week 8** | 14 miles<br>run 10 min/<br>walk 1 min<br>9:15–10:30 pace | off | 4 miles<br>tempo run<br>8:45 pace | 5 hills<br>85% effort<br>2 mi warm-up<br>2 mi cool-down | 4 miles<br>steady run<br>9:00 pace | 6 miles<br>fartlek<br>8:15–8:45 pace | 4 miles<br>steady<br>easy run |
| **Week 9** | 16 miles<br>run 10 min/<br>walk 1 min<br>9:15–10:30 pace | off | 6 miles<br>tempo run<br>8:45 pace | 6 hills<br>85% effort<br>2 mi warm-up<br>2 mi cool-down | 4 miles<br>steady run<br>9:00 pace | 6 miles<br>fartlek<br>8:15–8:45 pace | 4 miles<br>steady<br>easy run |

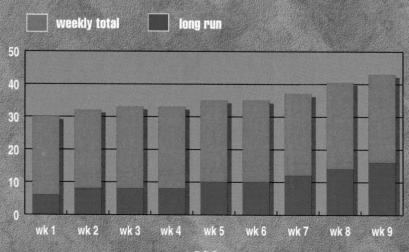

◻ weekly total    ◼ long run

## *miles*    3 hr. 45 min. marathon
### *training program*

| | SUN | MON | TUES | WED | THURS | FRI | SAT |
|---|---|---|---|---|---|---|---|
| **Week 10** | **12 miles** run 10 min/ walk 1 min 9:15–10:30 pace | off | **6 miles** tempo run 8:45 pace | **7 hills** 85% effort 2 mi warm-up 2 mi cool-down | **4 miles** steady run 9:00 pace | **6 miles** fartlek 8:15–8:45 pace | **4 miles** steady easy run |
| **Week 11** | **18 miles** run 10 min/ walk 1 min 9:15–10:30 pace | off | **4 miles** tempo run 8:45 pace | **8 hills** 85% effort 2 mi warm-up 2 mi cool-down | **5 miles** steady run 9:00 pace | **6 miles** fartlek 8:15–8:45 pace | **4 miles** steady easy run |
| **Week 12** | **18 miles** run 10 min/ walk 1 min 9:15–10:30 pace | off | **4 miles** tempo run 8:45 pace | **9 hills** 85% effort 2 mi warm-up 2 mi cool-down | **4 miles** steady run 9:00 pace | **6 miles** fartlek 8:15–8:45 pace | **4 miles** steady easy run |
| **Week 13** | **20 miles** run 10 min/ walk 1 min 9:15–10:30 pace | off | **4 miles** tempo run 8:45 pace | **10 hills** 85% effort 2 mi warm-up 2 mi cool-down | **4 miles** steady run 9:00 pace | **6 miles** fartlek 8:15–8:45 pace | **4 miles** steady easy run |
| **Week 14** | **14 miles** run 10 min/ walk 1 min 9:15–10:30 pace | off | **4 miles** tempo run 8:45 pace | **2 speed int.** 1 mi @ 7:20/mi 2 mi warm-up 2 mi cool-down | **5 miles** steady run 9:00 pace | **6 miles** fartlek 8:15–8:45 pace | **4 miles** steady easy run |
| **Week 15** | **18 miles** run 10 min/ walk 1 min 9:15–10:30 pace | off | **4 miles** tempo run 8:45 pace | **3 speed int.** 1 mi @ 7:20/mi 2 mi warm-up 2 mi cool-down | **4 miles** steady run 9:00 pace | **6 miles** fartlek 8:15–8:45 pace | **4 miles** steady easy run |
| **Week 16** | **20 miles** run 10 min/ walk 1 min 9:15–10:30 pace | off | **4 miles** tempo run 8:45 pace | **4 speed int.** 1 mi @ 7:20/mi 2 mi warm-up 2 mi cool-down | **4 miles** steady run 9:00 pace | **6 miles** fartlek 8:15–8:45 pace | **4 miles** steady easy run |
| **Week 17** | **14 miles** run 10 min/ walk 1 min 9:15–10:30 pace | off | **4 miles** tempo run 8:45 pace | **5 speed int.** 1 mi @ 7:20/mi 2 mi warm-up 2 mi cool-down | **4 miles** steady run 9:00 pace | **6 miles** fartlek 8:15–8:45 pace | **10 miles** race pace (8:35 pace) |
| **Week 18** | **4 miles** easy run 9:15–10:30 pace | off | **4 miles** race pace (8:35 pace) | **6 miles** race pace (8:35 pace) | off | off | **2 miles** steady easy run |
| **FINALE!** | **26 miles** RACE DAY! 8:35 pace | | | | | | |

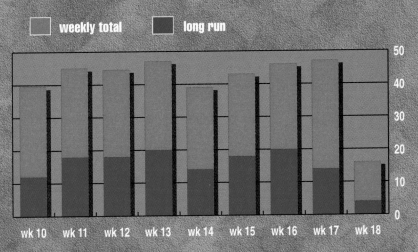

☐ **weekly total**    ■ **long run**

wk 10   wk 11   wk 12   wk 13   wk 14   wk 15   wk 16   wk 17   wk 18

# 3 hr. 30 min. marathon
*training program*

## kilometres

| | SUN | MON | TUES | WED | THURS | FRI | SAT |
|---|---|---|---|---|---|---|---|
| **Week 1** | **10 km** run 10 min/ walk 1 min 5:25–5:50 pace | off | **8 km** tempo run 5:10 pace | **10 km** steady run 5:15 pace | **10 km** fartlek 4:50–5:10 pace | **8 km** steady run 5:15 pace | **8 km** steady easy run |
| **Week 2** | **13 km** run 10 min/ walk 1 min 5:25–5:50 pace | off | **8 km** tempo run 5:10 pace | **10 km** steady run 5:15 pace | **10 km** fartlek 4:50–5:10 pace | **8 km** steady run 5:15 pace | **8 km** steady easy run |
| **Week 3** | **13 km** run 10 min/ walk 1 min 5:25–5:50 pace | off | **8 km** tempo run 5:10 pace | **10 km** steady run 5:15 pace | **10 km** fartlek 4:50–5:10 pace | **8 km** steady run 5:15 pace | **8 km** steady easy run |
| **Week 4** | **13 km** run 10 min/ walk 1 min 5:25–5:50 pace | off | **8 km** tempo run 5:10 pace | **10 km** steady run 5:15 pace | **10 km** fartlek 4:50–5:10 pace | **8 km** steady run 5:15 pace | **8 km** steady easy run |
| **Week 5** | **16 km** run 10 min/ walk 1 min 5:25–5:50 pace | off | **8 km** tempo run 5:10 pace | **10 km** steady run 5:15 pace | **10 km** fartlek 4:50–5:10 pace | **8 km** steady run 5:15 pace | **8 km** steady easy run |
| **Week 6** | **16 km** run 10 min/ walk 1 min 5:25–5:50 pace | off | **8 km** tempo run 5:10 pace | **10 km** steady run 5:15 pace | **10 km** fartlek 4:50–5:10 pace | **8 km** steady run 5:15 pace | **8 km** steady easy run |
| **Week 7** | **19 km** run 10 min/ walk 1 min 5:25–5:50 pace | off | **8 km** tempo run 5:10 pace | **4 hills** 85% effort 3 km warm-up 3 km cool-down | **8 km** steady run 5:15 pace | **10 km** fartlek 4:50–5:10 pace | **8 km** steady easy run |
| **Week 8** | **23 km** run 10 min/ walk 1 min 5:25–5:50 pace | off | **8 km** tempo run 5:10 pace | **5 hills** 85% effort 3 km warm-up 3 km cool-down | **8 km** steady run 5:15 pace | **10 km** fartlek 4:50–5:10 pace | **8 km** steady easy run |
| **Week 9** | **26 km** run 10 min/ walk 1 min 5:25–5:50 pace | off | **8 km** tempo run 5:10 pace | **6 hills** 85% effort 3 km warm-up 3 km cool-down | **8 km** steady run 5:15 pace | **10 km** fartlek 4:50–5:10 pace | **8 km** steady easy run |

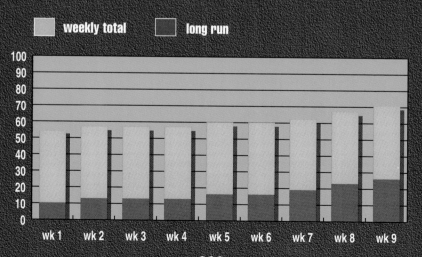

weekly total    long run

230

# *kilometres* — 3 hr. 30 min. marathon
### *training program*

| | SUN | MON | TUES | WED | THURS | FRI | SAT |
|---|---|---|---|---|---|---|---|
| **Week 10** | **19 km** run 10 min/ walk 1 min 5:25–5:50 pace | off | **8 km** tempo run 5:10 pace | **7 hills** 85% effort 3 km warm-up 3 km cool-down | **8 km** steady run 5:15 pace | **10 km** fartlek 4:50–5:10 pace | **8 km** steady easy run |
| **Week 11** | **29 km** run 10 min/ walk 1 min 5:25–5:50 pace | off | **8 km** tempo run 5:10 pace | **8 hills** 85% effort 3 km warm-up 3 km cool-down | **8 km** steady run 5:15 pace | **10 km** fartlek 4:50–5:10 pace | **8 km** steady easy run |
| **Week 12** | **29 km** run 10 min/ walk 1 min 5:25–5:50 pace | off | **8 km** tempo run 5:10 pace | **9 hills** 85% effort 3 km warm-up 3 km cool-down | **8 km** steady run 5:15 pace | **10 km** fartlek 4:50–5:10 pace | **8 km** steady easy run |
| **Week 13** | **32 km** run 10 min/ walk 1 min 5:25–5:50 pace | off | **8 km** tempo run 5:10 pace | **10 hills** 85% effort 3 km warm-up 3 km cool-down | **8 km** steady run 5:15 pace | **10 km** fartlek 4:50–5:10 pace | **8 km** steady easy run |
| **Week 14** | **22 km** run 10 min/ walk 1 min 5:25–5:50 pace | off | **8 km** tempo run 5:10 pace | **2 speed int.** 1.6 km @ 4:20/km 3 km warm-up 3 km cool-down | **8 km** steady run 5:15 pace | **10 km** fartlek 4:50–5:10 pace | **8 km** steady easy run |
| **Week 15** | **29 km** run 10 min/ walk 1 min 5:25–5:50 pace | off | **8 km** tempo run 5:10 pace | **3 speed int.** 1.6 km @ 4:20/km 3 km warm-up 3 km cool-down | **8 km** steady run 5:15 pace | **10 km** fartlek 4:50–5:10 pace | **8 km** steady easy run |
| **Week 16** | **32 km** run 10 min/ walk 1 min 5:25–5:50 pace | off | **8 km** tempo run 5:10 pace | **4 speed int.** 1.6 km @ 4:20/km 3 km warm-up 3 km cool-down | **8 km** steady run 5:15 pace | **10 km** fartlek 4:50–5:10 pace | **8 km** steady easy run |
| **Week 17** | **23 km** run 10 min/ walk 1 min 5:25–5:50 pace | off | **8 km** tempo run 5:10 pace | **5 speed int.** 1.6 km @ 4:20/km 3 km warm-up 3 km cool-down | **8 km** steady run 5:15 pace | **10 km** fartlek 4:50–5:10 pace | **16 km** race pace (5:00 pace) |
| **Week 18** | **6 km** easy run 5:25–5:50 pace | off | **8 km** race pace (5:00 pace) | **10 km** race pace (5:00 pace) | off | off | **3 km** steady easy run |
| **FINALE!** | **42 km** RACE DAY! 4:59 pace | | | | | | |

**weekly total**   **long run**

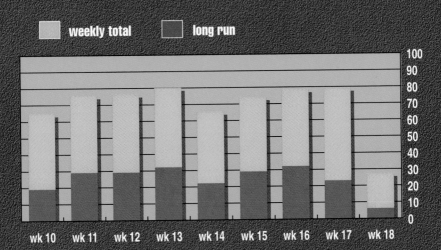

wk 10  wk 11  wk 12  wk 13  wk 14  wk 15  wk 16  wk 17  wk 18

100 90 80 70 60 50 40 30 20 10 0

# 3 hr. 30 min. marathon
## training program

*miles*

| | SUN | MON | TUES | WED | THURS | FRI | SAT |
|---|---|---|---|---|---|---|---|
| **Week 1** | **6 miles** run 10 min/ walk 1 min 8:45–10:00 pace | off | **5 miles** tempo run 8:20 pace | **6 miles** steady run 8:30 pace | **6 miles** fartlek 7:45–8:15 pace | **5 miles** steady run 8:30 pace | **5 miles** steady easy run |
| **Week 2** | **8 miles** run 10 min/ walk 1 min 8:45–10:00 pace | off | **5 miles** tempo run 8:20 pace | **6 miles** steady run 8:30 pace | **6 miles** fartlek 7:45–8:15 pace | **5 miles** steady run 8:30 pace | **5 miles** steady easy run |
| **Week 3** | **8 miles** run 10 min/ walk 1 min 8:45–10:00 pace | off | **5 miles** tempo run 8:20 pace | **6 miles** steady run 8:30 pace | **6 miles** fartlek 7:45–8:15 pace | **5 miles** steady run 8:30 pace | **5 miles** steady easy run |
| **Week 4** | **8 miles** run 10 min/ walk 1 min 8:45–10:00 pace | off | **5 miles** tempo run 8:20 pace | **6 miles** steady run 8:30 pace | **6 miles** fartlek 7:45–8:15 pace | **5 miles** steady run 8:30 pace | **5 miles** steady easy run |
| **Week 5** | **10 miles** run 10 min/ walk 1 min 8:45–10:00 pace | off | **5 miles** tempo run 8:20 pace | **6 miles** steady run 8:30 pace | **6 miles** fartlek 7:45–8:15 pace | **5 miles** steady run 8:30 pace | **5 miles** steady easy run |
| **Week 6** | **10 miles** run 10 min/ walk 1 min 8:45–10:00 pace | off | **5 miles** tempo run 8:20 pace | **6 miles** steady run 8:30 pace | **6 miles** fartlek 7:45–8:15 pace | **5 miles** steady run 8:30 pace | **5 miles** steady easy run |
| **Week 7** | **12 miles** run 10 min/ walk 1 min 8:45–10:00 pace | off | **5 miles** tempo run 8:20 pace | **4 hills** 85% effort 2 mi warm-up 2 mi cool-down | **5 miles** steady run 8:30 pace | **6 miles** fartlek 7:45–8:15 pace | **5 miles** steady easy run |
| **Week 8** | **14 miles** run 10 min/ walk 1 min 8:45–10:00 pace | off | **6 miles** tempo run 8:20 pace | **5 hills** 85% effort 2 mi warm-up 2 mi cool-down | **5 miles** steady run 8:30 pace | **6 miles** fartlek 7:45–8:15 pace | **5 miles** steady easy run |
| **Week 9** | **16 miles** run 10 min/ walk 1 min 8:45–10:00 pace | off | **5 miles** tempo run 8:20 pace | **6 hills** 85% effort 2 mi warm-up 2 mi cool-down | **5 miles** steady run 8:30 pace | **6 miles** fartlek 7:45–8:15 pace | **5 miles** steady easy run |

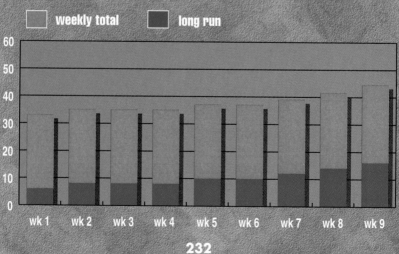

weekly total ▢    long run ▨

# 3 hr. 30 min. marathon

*training program*

| | SUN | MON | TUES | WED | THURS | FRI | SAT |
|---|---|---|---|---|---|---|---|
| **Week 10** | **12 miles** run 10 min/ walk 1 min 8:45–10:00 pace | off | **5 miles** tempo run 8:20 pace | **7 hills** 85% effort 2 mi warm-up 2 mi cool-down | **5 miles** steady run 8:30 pace | **6 miles** fartlek 7:45–8:15 pace | **5 miles** steady easy run |
| **Week 11** | **18 miles** run 10 min/ walk 1 min 8:45–10:00 pace | off | **5 miles** tempo run 8:20 pace | **8 hills** 85% effort 2 mi warm-up 2 mi cool-down | **5 miles** steady run 8:30 pace | **6 miles** fartlek 7:45–8:15 pace | **5 miles** steady easy run |
| **Week 12** | **18 miles** run 10 min/ walk 1 min 8:45–10:00 pace | off | **5 miles** tempo run 8:20 pace | **9 hills** 85% effort 2 mi warm-up 2 mi cool-down | **5 miles** steady run 8:30 pace | **6 miles** fartlek 7:45–8:15 pace | **5 miles** steady easy run |
| **Week 13** | **20 miles** run 10 min/ walk 1 min 8:45–10:00 pace | off | **5 miles** tempo run 8:20 pace | **10 hills** 85% effort 2 mi warm-up 2 mi cool-down | **5 miles** steady run 8:30 pace | **6 miles** fartlek 7:45–8:15 pace | **5 miles** steady easy run |
| **Week 14** | **14 miles** run 10 min/ walk 1 min 8:45–10:00 pace | off | **5 miles** tempo run 8:20 pace | **2 speed int.** 1 mi @ 7:00/mi 2 mi warm-up 2 mi cool-down | **5 miles** steady run 8:30 pace | **6 miles** fartlek 7:45–8:15 pace | **5 miles** steady easy run |
| **Week 15** | **18 miles** run 10 min/ walk 1 min 8:45–10:00 pace | off | **5 miles** tempo run 8:20 pace | **3 speed int.** 1 mi @ 7:00/mi 2 mi warm-up 2 mi cool-down | **5 miles** steady run 8:30 pace | **6 miles** fartlek 7:45–8:15 pace | **5 miles** steady easy run |
| **Week 16** | **20 miles** run 10 min/ walk 1 min 8:45–10:00 pace | off | **5 miles** tempo run 8:20 pace | **4 speed int.** 1 mi @ 7:00/mi 2 mi warm-up 2 mi cool-down | **5 miles** steady run 8:30 pace | **6 miles** fartlek 7:45–8:15 pace | **5 miles** steady easy run |
| **Week 17** | **14 miles** run 10 min/ walk 1 min 8:45–10:00 pace | off | **5 miles** tempo run 8:20 pace | **5 speed int.** 1 mi @ 7:00/mi 2 mi warm-up 2 mi cool-down | **5 miles** steady run 8:30 pace | **6 miles** fartlek 7:45–8:15 pace | **10 miles** race pace (8:00 pace) |
| **Week 18** | **4 miles** steady run 8:45–10:00 pace | off | **5 miles** race pace (8:00 pace) | **6 miles** race pace (8:00 pace) | off | off | **2 miles** steady easy run |
| **FINALE!** | **26 miles** RACE DAY! 8:01 pace | | | | | | |

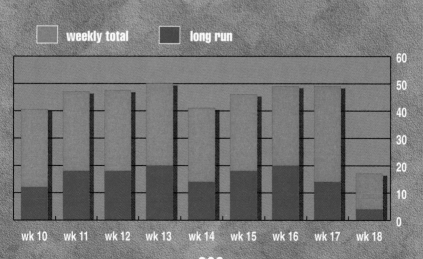

■ weekly total　■ long run

wk 10　wk 11　wk 12　wk 13　wk 14　wk 15　wk 16　wk 17　wk 18

60 50 40 30 20 10 0

# 3 hr. 10 min. marathon
*training program*

*kilometres*

| | SUN | MON | TUES | WED | THURS | FRI | SAT |
|---|---|---|---|---|---|---|---|
| **Week 1** | **10 km** steady run 5:00–5:35 pace | off | **8 km** tempo run 4:40 pace | **10 km** steady run 5:00 pace | **13 km** fartlek 4:20–4:50 pace | **13 km** steady run 5:00 pace | **8 km** steady easy run |
| **Week 2** | **13 km** steady run 5:00–5:35 pace | off | **8 km** tempo run 4:40 pace | **10 km** steady run 5:00 pace | **13 km** fartlek 4:20–4:50 pace | **13 km** steady run 5:00 pace | **8 km** steady easy run |
| **Week 3** | **16 km** steady run 5:00–5:35 pace | off | **8 km** tempo run 4:40 pace | **10 km** steady run 5:00 pace | **13 km** fartlek 4:20–4:50 pace | **13 km** steady run 5:00 pace | **8 km** steady easy run |
| **Week 4** | **16 km** steady run 5:00–5:35 pace | off | **8 km** tempo run 4:40 pace | **10 km** steady run 5:00 pace | **13 km** fartlek 4:20–4:50 pace | **13 km** steady run 5:00 pace | **8 km** steady easy run |
| **Week 5** | **19 km** steady run 5:00–5:35 pace | off | **8 km** tempo run 5:00 pace | **10 km** steady run 5:00 pace | **13 km** fartlek 4:20–4:50 pace | **13 km** steady run 5:00 pace | **8 km** steady easy run |
| **Week 6** | **23 km** steady run 5:00–5:35 pace | off | **8 km** tempo run 4:40 pace | **10 km** steady run 5:00 pace | **13 km** fartlek 4:20–4:50 pace | **13 km** steady run 5:00 pace | **8 km** steady easy run |
| **Week 7** | **26 km** steady run 5:00–5:35 pace | off | **8 km** tempo run 4:40 pace | **4 hills** 85% effort 3 km warm-up 3 km cool-down | **8 km** steady run 5:00 pace | **13 km** fartlek 4:20–4:50 pace | **8 km** steady easy run |
| **Week 8** | **26 km** steady run 5:00–5:35 pace | off | **11 km** tempo run 4:40 pace | **5 hills** 85% effort 3 km warm-up 3 km cool-down | **8 km** steady run 5:00 pace | **13 km** fartlek 4:20–4:50 pace | **8 km** steady easy run |
| **Week 9** | **22 km** steady run 5:00–5:35 pace | off | **11 km** tempo run 4:40 pace | **6 hills** 85% effort 3 km warm-up 3 km cool-down | **8 km** steady run 5:00 pace | **13 km** fartlek 4:20–4:50 pace | **8 km** steady easy run |

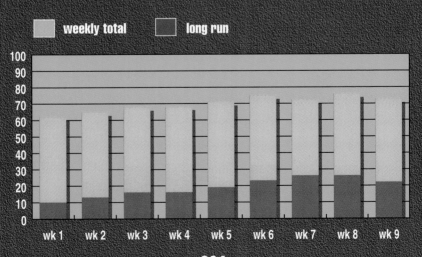

weekly total    long run

| | SUN | MON | TUES | WED | THURS | FRI | SAT |
|---|---|---|---|---|---|---|---|
| **Week 10** | 22 km steady run 5:00–5:35 pace | off | 11 km tempo run 4:40 pace | 7 hills 85% effort 3 km warm-up 3 km cool-down | 8 km steady run 5:00 pace | 13 km fartlek 4:20–4:50 pace | 8 km steady easy run |
| **Week 11** | 29 km steady run 5:00–5:35 pace | off | 8 km tempo run 4:40 pace | 8 hills 85% effort 3 km warm-up 3 km cool-down | 8 km steady run 5:00 pace | 13 km fartlek 4:20–4:50 pace | 8 km steady easy run |
| **Week 12** | 32 km steady run 5:00–5:35 pace | off | 8 km tempo run 4:40 pace | 9 hills 85% effort 3 km warm-up 3 km cool-down | 8 km steady run 5:00 pace | 13 km fartlek 4:20–4:50 pace | 8 km steady easy run |
| **Week 13** | 32 km steady run 5:00–5:35 pace | off | 8 km tempo run 4:40 pace | 10 hills 85% effort 3 km warm-up 3 km cool-down | 8 km steady run 5:00 pace | 13 km fartlek 4:20–4:50 pace | 8 km steady easy run |
| **Week 14** | 22 km steady run 5:00–5:35 pace | off | 8 km tempo run 4:40 pace | 2 speed int. 1.6 km @ 4:00/km 3 km warm-up 3 km cool-down | 8 km steady run 5:00 pace | 13 km fartlek 4:20–4:50 pace | 8 km steady easy run |
| **Week 15** | 32 km steady run 5:00–5:35 pace | off | 8 km tempo run 4:40 pace | 3 speed int. 1.6 km @ 4:00/km 3 km warm-up 3 km cool-down | 8 km steady run 5:00 pace | 13 km fartlek 4:20–4:50 pace | 8 km steady easy run |
| **Week 16** | 32 km steady run 5:00–5:35 pace | off | 8 km tempo run 4:40 pace | 4 speed int. 1.6 km @ 4:00/km 3 km warm-up 3 km cool-down | 8 km steady run 5:00 pace | 13 km fartlek 4:20–4:50 pace | 8 km steady easy run |
| **Week 17** | 22 km steady run 5:00–5:35 pace | off | 8 km tempo run 4:40 pace | 5 speed int. 1.6 km @ 4:00/km 3 km warm-up 3 km cool-down | 8 km steady run 5:00 pace | 13 km fartlek 4:20–4:50 pace | 16 km race pace (4:30 pace) |
| **Week 18** | 6 km steady run 5:00–5:35 pace | off | 8 km race pace (4:30 pace) | 10 km race pace (4:30 pace) | off | off | 3 km steady easy run |
| **FINALE!** | 42 km RACE DAY! 4:30 pace | | | | | | |

**weekly total**   **long run**

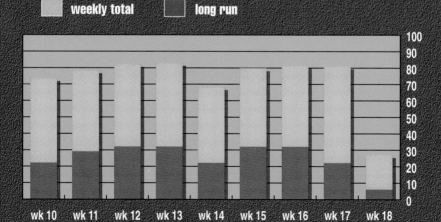

wk 10 · wk 11 · wk 12 · wk 13 · wk 14 · wk 15 · wk 16 · wk 17 · wk 18

100 90 80 70 60 50 40 30 20 10 0

# 3 hr. 10 min. marathon
## training program

*miles*

| | SUN | MON | TUES | WED | THURS | FRI | SAT |
|---|---|---|---|---|---|---|---|
| **Week 1** | **6 miles** steady run 8:00–9:00 pace | off | **5 miles** tempo run 7:30 pace | **6 miles** steady run 8:00 pace | **8 miles** fartlek 7:00–7:45 pace | **8 miles** steady run 8:00 pace | **5 miles** steady easy run |
| **Week 2** | **8 miles** steady run 8:00–9:00 pace | off | **5 miles** tempo run 7:30 pace | **6 miles** steady run 8:00 pace | **8 miles** fartlek 7:00–7:45 pace | **8 miles** steady run 8:00 pace | **5 miles** steady easy run |
| **Week 3** | **10 miles** steady run 8:00–9:00 pace | off | **5 miles** tempo run 7:30 pace | **6 miles** steady run 8:00 pace | **8 miles** fartlek 7:00–7:45 pace | **8 miles** steady run 8:00 pace | **5 miles** steady easy run |
| **Week 4** | **10 miles** steady run 8:00–9:00 pace | off | **5 miles** tempo run 7:30 pace | **6 miles** steady run 8:00 pace | **8 miles** fartlek 7:00–7:45 pace | **8 miles** steady run 8:00 pace | **5 miles** steady easy run |
| **Week 5** | **12 miles** steady run 8:00–9:00 pace | off | **5 miles** tempo run 7:30 pace | **6 miles** steady run 8:00 pace | **8 miles** fartlek 7:00–7:45 pace | **8 miles** steady run 8:00 pace | **5 miles** steady easy run |
| **Week 6** | **14 miles** steady run 8:00–9:00 pace | off | **5 miles** tempo run 7:30 pace | **6 miles** steady run 8:00 pace | **8 miles** fartlek 7:00–7:45 pace | **8 miles** steady run 8:00 pace | **5 miles** steady easy run |
| **Week 7** | **16 miles** steady run 8:00–9:00 pace | off | **5 miles** tempo run 7:30 pace | **4 hills** 85% effort 2 mi warm-up 2 mi cool-down | **5 miles** steady run 8:00 pace | **8 miles** fartlek 7:00–7:45 pace | **5 miles** steady easy run |
| **Week 8** | **16 miles** steady run 8:00–9:00 pace | off | **7 miles** tempo run 7:30 pace | **5 hills** 85% effort 2 mi warm-up 2 mi cool-down | **5 miles** steady run 8:00 pace | **8 miles** fartlek 7:00–7:45 pace | **5 miles** steady easy run |
| **Week 9** | **18 miles** steady run 8:00–9:00 pace | off | **7 miles** tempo run 7:30 pace | **6 hills** 85% effort 2 mi warm-up 2 mi cool-down | **5 miles** steady run 8:00 pace | **6 miles** fartlek 7:00–7:45 pace | **5 miles** steady easy run |

☐ weekly total   ☐ long run

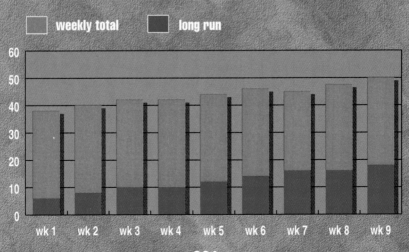

# 3 hr. 10 min. marathon
*training program*

| | SUN | MON | TUES | WED | THURS | FRI | SAT |
|---|---|---|---|---|---|---|---|
| **Week 10** | 14 miles<br>steady run<br>8:00–9:00 pace | off | 7 miles<br>tempo run<br>7:30 pace | 7 hills<br>85% effort<br>2 mi warm-up<br>2 mi cool-down | 5 miles<br>steady run<br>8:00 pace | 8 miles<br>fartlek<br>7:00–7:45 pace | 5 miles<br>steady<br>easy run |
| **Week 11** | 18 miles<br>steady run<br>8:00–9:00 pace | off | 5 miles<br>tempo run<br>7:30 pace | 8 hills<br>85% effort<br>2 mi warm-up<br>2 mi cool-down | 5 miles<br>steady run<br>8:00 pace | 8 miles<br>fartlek<br>7:00–7:45 pace | 5 miles<br>steady<br>easy run |
| **Week 12** | 20 miles<br>steady run<br>8:00–9:00 pace | off | 5 miles<br>tempo run<br>7:30 pace | 9 hills<br>85% effort<br>2 mi warm-up<br>2 mi cool-down | 5 miles<br>steady run<br>8:00 pace | 8 miles<br>fartlek<br>7:00–7:45 pace | 5 miles<br>steady<br>easy run |
| **Week 13** | 20 miles<br>steady run<br>8:00–9:00 pace | off | 5 miles<br>tempo run<br>7:30 pace | 10 hills<br>85% effort<br>2 mi warm-up<br>2 mi cool-down | 5 miles<br>steady run<br>8:00 pace | 8 miles<br>fartlek<br>7:00–7:45 pace | 5 miles<br>steady<br>easy run |
| **Week 14** | 14 miles<br>steady run<br>8:00–9:00 pace | off | 5 miles<br>tempo run<br>7:30 pace | 2 speed int.<br>1 mi @ 6:25/mi<br>2 mi warm-up<br>2 mi cool-down | 5 miles<br>steady run<br>8:00 pace | 8 miles<br>fartlek<br>7:00–7:45 pace | 5 miles<br>steady<br>easy run |
| **Week 15** | 20 miles<br>steady run<br>8:00–9:00 pace | off | 5 miles<br>tempo run<br>7:30 pace | 3 speed int.<br>1 mi @ 6:25/mi<br>2 mi warm-up<br>2 mi cool-down | 5 miles<br>steady run<br>8:00 pace | 8 miles<br>fartlek<br>7:00–7:45 pace | 5 miles<br>steady<br>easy run |
| **Week 16** | 20 miles<br>steady run<br>8:00–9:00 pace | off | 5 miles<br>tempo run<br>7:30 pace | 4 speed int.<br>1 mi @ 6:25/mi<br>2 mi warm-up<br>2 mi cool-down | 5 miles<br>steady run<br>8:00 pace | 8 miles<br>fartlek<br>7:00–7:45 pace | 5 miles<br>steady<br>easy run |
| **Week 17** | 14 miles<br>steady run<br>8:00–9:00 pace | off | 5 miles<br>tempo run<br>7:30 pace | 5 speed int.<br>1 mi @ 6:25/mi<br>2 mi warm-up<br>2 mi cool-down | 5 miles<br>steady run<br>8:00 pace | 8 miles<br>fartlek<br>7:00–7:45 pace | 10 miles<br>race pace<br>(7:15 pace) |
| **Week 18** | 4 miles<br>steady run<br>8:00–9:00 pace | off | 5 miles<br>race pace<br>(7:15 pace) | 6 miles<br>race pace<br>(7:15 pace) | off | off | 2 miles<br>steady<br>easy run |
| **FINALE!** | 26 miles<br>RACE DAY!<br>7:15 pace | | | | | | |

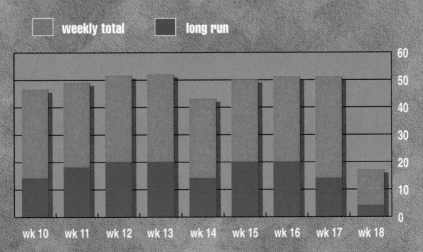

weekly total   long run

wk 10   wk 11   wk 12   wk 13   wk 14   wk 15   wk 16   wk 17   wk 18

# 3 hr. marathon
## training program
### kilometres

| | SUN | MON | TUES | WED | THURS | FRI | SAT |
|---|---|---|---|---|---|---|---|
| **Week 1** | **16 km** steady run 4:30–5:15 pace | off | **13 km** tempo run 4:20 pace | **10 km** steady run 4:40 pace | **13 km** fartlek 4:05–4:25 pace | **13 km** steady run 4:40 pace | **8 km** steady run 4:40 pace |
| **Week 2** | **16 km** steady run 4:30–5:15 pace | **8 km** steady easy run | **13 km** tempo run 4:20 pace | **10 km** steady run 4:40 pace | **13 km** fartlek 4:05–4:25 pace | **13 km** steady run 4:40 pace | **8 km** steady run 4:40 pace |
| **Week 3** | **19 km** steady run 4:30–5:15 pace | **8 km** steady easy run | **13 km** tempo run 4:20 pace | **10 km** steady run 4:40 pace | **13 km** fartlek 4:05–4:25 pace | **13 km** steady run 4:40 pace | **8 km** steady run 4:40 pace |
| **Week 4** | **19 km** steady run 4:30–5:15 pace | off | **13 km** tempo run 4:20 pace | **4 hills** 85% effort 3 km warm-up 3 km cool-down | **8 km** steady run 4:40 pace | **13 km** fartlek 4:05–4:25 pace | **8 km** steady run 4:40 pace |
| **Week 5** | **22 km** steady run 4:30–5:15 pace | **8 km** steady easy run | **13 km** tempo run 4:20 pace | **5 hills** 85% effort 3 km warm-up 3 km cool-down | **8 km** steady run 4:40 pace | **13 km** fartlek 4:05–4:25 pace | **8 km** steady run 4:40 pace |
| **Week 6** | **22 km** steady run 4:30–5:15 pace | **8 km** steady easy run | **13 km** tempo run 4:20 pace | **5 hills** 85% effort 3 km warm-up 3 km cool-down | **8 km** steady run 4:40 pace | **13 km** fartlek 4:05–4:25 pace | **8 km** steady run 4:40 pace |
| **Week 7** | **26 km** steady run 4:30–5:15 pace | off | **13 km** tempo run 4:20 pace | **6 hills** 85% effort 3 km warm-up 3 km cool-down | **8 km** steady run 4:40 pace | **13 km** fartlek 4:05–4:25 pace | **8 km** steady run 4:40 pace |
| **Week 8** | **29 km** steady run 4:30–5:15 pace | **8 km** steady easy run | **13 km** tempo run 4:20 pace | **6 hills** 85% effort 3 km warm-up 3 km cool-down | **8 km** steady run 4:40 pace | **13 km** fartlek 4:05–4:25 pace | **8 km** steady run 4:40 pace |
| **Week 9** | **22 km** steady run 4:30–5:15 pace | **8 km** steady easy run | **13 km** tempo run 4:20 pace | **7 hills** 85% effort 3 km warm-up 3 km cool-down | **8 km** steady run 4:40 pace | **13 km** fartlek 4:05–4:25 pace | **8 km** steady run 4:40 pace |

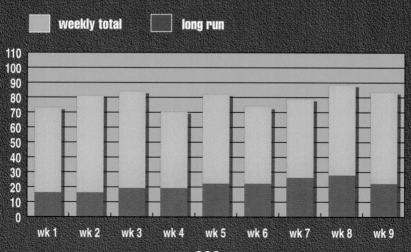

weekly total    long run

# kilometres

# 3 hr. marathon
## training program

| | SUN | MON | TUES | WED | THURS | FRI | SAT |
|---|---|---|---|---|---|---|---|
| **Week 10** | 29 km<br>steady run<br>4:30–5:15 pace | off | 13 km<br>tempo run<br>4:20 pace | 7 hills<br>85% effort<br>3 km warm-up<br>3 km cool-down | 8 km<br>steady run<br>4:40 pace | 13 km<br>fartlek<br>4:05–4:25 pace | 8 km<br>steady run<br>4:40 pace |
| **Week 11** | 32 km<br>steady run<br>4:30–5:15 pace | 8 km<br>steady<br>easy run | 13 km<br>tempo run<br>4:20 pace | 8 hills<br>85% effort<br>3 km warm-up<br>3 km cool-down | 8 km<br>steady run<br>4:40 pace | 13 km<br>fartlek<br>4:05–4:25 pace | 8 km<br>steady run<br>4:40 pace |
| **Week 12** | 32 km<br>steady run<br>4:30–5:15 pace | 8 km<br>steady<br>easy run | 13 km<br>tempo run<br>4:20 pace | 9 hills<br>85% effort<br>3 km warm-up<br>3 km cool-down | 8 km<br>steady run<br>4:40 pace | 13 km<br>fartlek<br>4:05–4:25 pace | 8 km<br>steady run<br>4:40 pace |
| **Week 13** | 32 km<br>steady run<br>4:30–5:15 pace | 8 km<br>steady<br>easy run | 13 km<br>tempo run<br>4:20 pace | 10 hills<br>85% effort<br>3 km warm-up<br>3 km cool-down | 8 km<br>steady run<br>4:40 pace | 13 km<br>fartlek<br>4:05–4:25 pace | 8 km<br>steady run<br>4:40 pace |
| **Week 14** | 22 km<br>steady run<br>4:30–5:15 pace | 8 km<br>steady<br>easy run | 13 km<br>tempo run<br>4:20 pace | 2 speed int.<br>1.6 km @ 3:50/km<br>3 km warm-up<br>3 km cool-down | 8 km<br>steady run<br>4:40 pace | 13 km<br>fartlek<br>4:05–4:25 pace | 8 km<br>steady run<br>4:40 pace |
| **Week 15** | 32 km<br>steady run<br>4:30–5:15 pace | 8 km<br>steady<br>easy run | 13 km<br>tempo run<br>4:20 pace | 3 speed int.<br>1.6 km @ 3:50/km<br>3 km warm-up<br>3 km cool-down | 8 km<br>steady run<br>4:40 pace | 13 km<br>fartlek<br>4:05–4:25 pace | 8 km<br>steady run<br>4:40 pace |
| **Week 16** | 32 km<br>steady run<br>4:30–5:15 pace | 8 km<br>steady<br>easy run | 13 km<br>tempo run<br>4:20 pace | 4 speed int.<br>1.6 km @ 3:50/km<br>3 km warm-up<br>3 km cool-down | 8 km<br>steady run<br>4:40 pace | 13 km<br>fartlek<br>4:05–4:25 pace | 8 km<br>steady run<br>4:40 pace |
| **Week 17** | 23 km<br>steady run<br>4:30–5:15 pace | 8 km<br>steady<br>easy run | 13 km<br>tempo run<br>4:20 pace | 5 speed int.<br>1.6 km @ 3:50/km<br>3 km warm-up<br>3 km cool-down | 8 km<br>steady run<br>4:40 pace | 13 km<br>fartlek<br>4:05–4:25 pace | 16 km<br>race pace<br>(4:15 pace) |
| **Week 18** | 6 km<br>steady run<br>4:30–5:15 pace | off | 13 km<br>race pace<br>(4:15 pace) | 10 km<br>race pace<br>(4:15 pace) | off | off | 3 km<br>steady<br>easy run |
| **FINALE!** | 42 km<br>RACE DAY!<br>4:16 pace | | | | | | |

*am*

■ weekly total   ■ long run

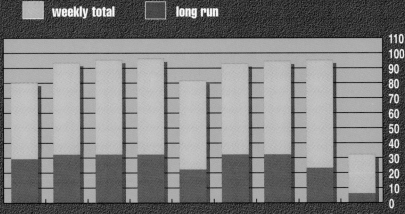

# 3 hr. marathon

*training program*

*miles*

| | SUN | MON | TUES | WED | THURS | FRI | SAT |
|---|---|---|---|---|---|---|---|
| **Week 1** | **10 miles** steady run 7:30–8:30 pace | off | **8 miles** tempo run 7:00 pace | **6 miles** steady run 7:30 pace | **8 miles** fartlek 6:35–7:05 pace | **8 miles** steady run 7:30 pace | **5 miles** steady run 7:30 pace |
| **Week 2** | **10 miles** steady run 7:30–8:30 pace | **5 miles** steady easy run | **8 miles** tempo run 7:00 pace | **6 miles** steady run 7:30 pace | **8 miles** fartlek 6:35–7:05 pace | **8 miles** steady run 7:30 pace | **5 miles** steady run 7:30 pace |
| **Week 3** | **12 miles** steady run 7:30–8:30 pace | **5 miles** steady easy run | **8 miles** tempo run 7:00 pace | **6 miles** steady run 7:30 pace | **8 miles** fartlek 6:35–7:05 pace | **8 miles** steady run 7:30 pace | **5 miles** steady run 7:30 pace |
| **Week 4** | **12 miles** steady run 7:30–8:30 pace | off | **8 miles** tempo run 7:00 pace | **4 hills** 85% effort 2 mi warm-up 2 mi cool-down | **5 miles** steady run 7:30 pace | **8 miles** fartlek 6:35–7:05 pace | **5 miles** steady run 7:30 pace |
| **Week 5** | **14 miles** steady run 7:30–8:30 pace | **5 miles** steady easy run | **8 miles** tempo run 7:00 pace | **5 hills** 85% effort 2 mi warm-up 2 mi cool-down | **5 miles** steady run 7:30 pace | **8 miles** fartlek 6:35–7:05 pace | **5 miles** steady run 7:30 pace |
| **Week 6** | **14 miles** steady run 7:30–8:30 pace | **5 miles** steady easy run | **8 miles** tempo run 7:00 pace | **5 hills** 85% effort 2 mi warm-up 2 mi cool-down | **5 miles** steady run 7:30 pace | **8 miles** fartlek 6:35–7:05 pace | **5 miles** steady run 7:30 pace |
| **Week 7** | **16 miles** steady run 7:30–8:30 pace | off | **8 miles** tempo run 7:00 pace | **6 hills** 85% effort 2 mi warm-up 2 mi cool-down | **5 miles** steady run 7:30 pace | **8 miles** fartlek 6:35–7:05 pace | **5 miles** steady run 7:30 pace |
| **Week 8** | **18 miles** steady run 7:30–8:30 pace | **5 miles** steady easy run | **8 miles** tempo run 7:00 pace | **6 hills** 85% effort 2 mi warm-up 2 mi cool-down | **5 miles** steady run 7:30 pace | **8 miles** fartlek 6:35–7:05 pace | **5 miles** steady run 7:30 pace |
| **Week 9** | **14 miles** steady run 7:30–8:30 pace | **5 miles** steady easy run | **8 miles** tempo run 7:00 pace | **7 hills** 85% effort 2 mi warm-up 2 mi cool-down | **5 miles** steady run 7:30 pace | **8 miles** fartlek 6:35–7:05 pace | **5 miles** steady run 7:30 pace |

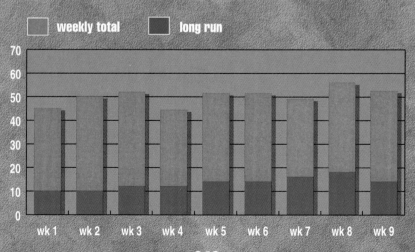

weekly total ◻   long run ◼

240

# miles

# 3 hr. marathon
### training program

| | SUN | MON | TUES | WED | THURS | FRI | SAT |
|---|---|---|---|---|---|---|---|
| **Week 10** | 18 miles steady run 7:30–8:30 pace | off | 8 miles tempo run 7:00 pace | 7 hills 85% effort 2 mi warm-up 2 mi cool-down | 5 miles steady run 7:30 pace | 8 miles fartlek 6:35–7:05 pace | 5 miles steady run 7:30 pace |
| **Week 11** | 20 miles steady run 7:30–8:30 pace | 5 miles easy run | 8 miles tempo run 7:00 pace | 8 hills 85% effort 2 mi warm-up 2 mi cool-down | 5 miles steady run 7:30 pace | 8 miles fartlek 6:35–7:05 pace | 5 miles steady run 7:30 pace |
| **Week 12** | 20 miles steady run 7:30–8:30 pace | 5 miles steady easy run | 8 miles tempo run 7:00 pace | 9 hills 85% effort 2 mi warm-up 2 mi cool-down | 5 miles steady run 7:30 pace | 8 miles fartlek 6:35–7:05 pace | 5 miles steady run 7:30 pace |
| **Week 13** | 20 miles steady run 7:30–8:30 pace | 5 miles steady easy run | 8 miles tempo run 7:00 pace | 10 hills 85% effort 2 mi warm-up 2 mi cool-down | 5 miles steady run 7:30 pace | 8 miles fartlek 6:35–7:05 pace | 5 miles steady run 7:30 pace |
| **Week 14** | 16 miles steady run 7:30–8:30 pace | 5 miles steady easy run | 8 miles tempo run 7:00 pace | 2 speed int. 1 mi @ 6:10/mi 2 mi warm-up 2 mi cool-down | 5 miles steady run 7:30 pace | 8 miles fartlek 6:35–7:05 pace | 5 miles steady run 7:30 pace |
| **Week 15** | 20 miles steady run 7:30–8:30 pace | 5 miles steady easy run | 8 miles tempo run 7:00 pace | 3 speed int. 1 mi @ 6:10/mi 2 mi warm-up 2 mi cool-down | 5 miles steady run 7:30 pace | 8 miles fartlek 6:35–7:05 pace | 5 miles steady run 7:30 pace |
| **Week 16** | 20 miles steady run 7:30–8:30 pace | 5 miles steady easy run | 8 miles tempo run 7:00 pace | 4 speed int. 1 mi @ 6:10/mi 2 mi warm-up 2 mi cool-down | 5 miles steady run 7:30 pace | 8 miles fartlek 6:35–7:05 pace | 5 miles steady easy run |
| **Week 17** | 14 miles steady run 7:30–8:30 pace | 5 miles steady easy run | 8 miles tempo run 7:00 pace | 5 speed int. 1 mi @ 6:10/mi 2 mi warm-up 2 mi cool-down | 5 miles steady run 7:30 pace | 8 miles fartlek 6:35–7:05 pace | 10 miles race pace (6:50 pace) |
| **Week 18** | 4 miles steady run 7:30–8:30 pace | off | 8 miles race pace (6:50 pace) | 6 miles race pace (6:50 pace) | off | off | 2 miles steady easy run |
| **FINALE!** | 26 miles RACE DAY! 6:52 pace | | | | | | |

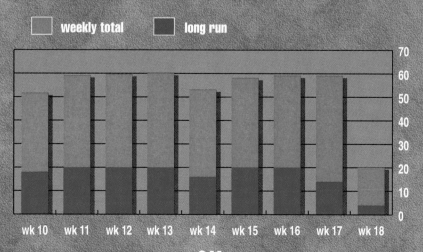

- weekly total
- long run

70
60
50
40
30
20
10
0

wk 10    wk 11    wk 12    wk 13    wk 14    wk 15    wk 16    wk 17    wk 18

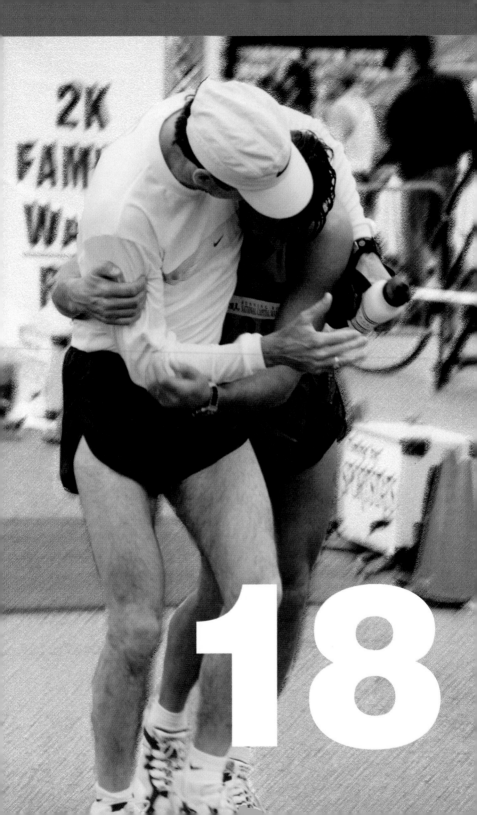

18

# Race Tips

Racing should be a memorable experience that stimulates you to test your training. Always keep things in perspective, and let common sense prevail—if anything out of your control goes wrong, you can always race again.

Some folks race to see if the hard work of their training and any modifications they made to their program are working. Friendly competition amongst training buddies is also a frequent race day test, whether they train at a 6-minute pace or a 10-minute pace. Many of us are at the races for the social aspect—we are infected with the positive energy that comes from the crowd at the start and the finish line. The laughter and camaraderie inspires us to perform and gives us a sense of renewal to take back to our daily training.

Some race directors even use their post-race goodies to draw folks out to the race. The popularity of the bagel has improved the post-race food selection from the traditional cookie and muffin; however, who can say no to chocolate chip cookies after a run?

Now that we have you in race mood, thinking about cookies, fun people and running a little faster, let's look at some ways to make the build-up to the race, the race itself and the day after the race a little more beneficial and enjoyable.

## The Build-up

### The Week Before

The week leading into a race should generally be a time of tapering off your mileage and resting. It is not the time to get into a race with a training buddy—save the challenges for race day. The sports medicine folks will tell you that there is a two-week training effect—most of what we do today takes two weeks to have an effect on our training—so nothing you do in the final week can have a positive effect on your race performance. Overtraining or risking injury in the final week, however, can certainly have a negative effect.

During the final week leading into the race, you should concentrate on keeping yourself well hydrated with water, eating a high balance of complex carbohydrates and limiting the amount of fat in your diet. I also recommend that you don't have any alcoholic drinks this week; replace them with water or fruit juice. It isn't that many runners don't enjoy an occasional cold beer or glass of fine

CH. 18

wine, but alcohol acts as a diuretic, which can cause you to lose precious water. Save the alcohol for after the run; it can be used then to treat yourself for a fine performance.

Two days before the race is the key time to get some extra sleep to insure that you are coming into the race well rested and not fatigued, especially if you are travelling to a race away from home. Continue to drink a lot of water, eat complex carbohydrates and avoid too much fat. It is also a good day to relax with some friends over supper. Try to eat relatively early, and then head home to relax and get an early sleep. If at all possible, don't set an alarm for the next morning—get as much sleep as possible.

## The Day Before

Water is the word of the day. Carry a water bottle with you everywhere you go and drink as much as you can. Your performance will improve through proper hydration, and you can't drink too much—frequent trips to the washroom are a good sign that you are indeed well hydrated. Try to drink 6 ounces (170 ml) of water every hour. Your urine will be almost colourless if you are drinking enough. Don't worry, there are always portable toilets at the race site. Nervousness will sometimes create the sensation of having to urinate, but after one trip you will usually be convinced that you don't really need to go again.

Your first meal of the day should be a high-carbohydrate breakfast. Each of us has an individual favourite. Mine is pancakes—hold the bacon and bring on the side order of toast. A low-fat sandwich makes a good lunch, and fresh fruit is great to snack on throughout the day. Try to eat early in the evening, if your schedule allows it, and eat a moderate portion. Do not try to carbohydrate load—all you will do is over-eat and be left feeling heavy and sluggish for the race. Some of the carbohydrate drinks are easier to digest than solid foods, but they lack the satisfaction that comes with a meal. The night before a race is not the time to try any new exotic foods. Go with a meal you used in training that left you feeling the best in your training runs.

Many times, folks will enter a race away from home. Travel is a fun way to involve the non-running folks in your life in your running and to give you a target to shoot for during your training. Be careful not to spend the day before the race walking around touring; it can leave your legs feeling like you have already run the race.

Pick up your race package the day before to avoid any last minute line-ups and tension on race morning. Double-check the start time, location and parking, and have a clear idea about how to get to the start line in a comfortable, non-stressed manner. Races are fun. They are part of your play time, so no stress should be allowed. The good folks that organize the events are for the most part

**CH. 18**

volunteers that are there because they share your passion for running because of the great causes that many races and fun runs assist. I say this so we all remember it when we are faced with the odd glitch that can come in when organizing these events.

Race package pick-up areas can be fun spots to be around. Just remember to limit your time to a good shot of enthusiasm. Hanging around too long can leave you tired, so head home or back to your hotel to review all of your gear for the race. When you have all your gear in order, the best place to be is in a prone position. Stay relaxed. Some folks find that their favourite music, a good movie or a favourite book is a good way to relax. I find that red licorice or a couple of chocolate chip cookies are good treats to munch on the evening before the race. The licorice is sweet, yet low in fat, and chewy, so enjoy; just don't eat the whole bag.

Once you are comfortable, start your race visualization, which will prepare you for the event the next day (see chapter 19 [Mental Preparation]). Plan for success and you will succeed. It's simple, so relax and enjoy.

During the night, you may find yourself up going to the washroom because of the great hydration you have done in the past 24 hours. Don't worry about the lack of sleep. Folks are often nervous and sleep doesn't come easily, so look at it this way: being well hydrated gives you something to do all night. Your good sleep of two nights before, combined with the training taper, is what will pay off during the race.

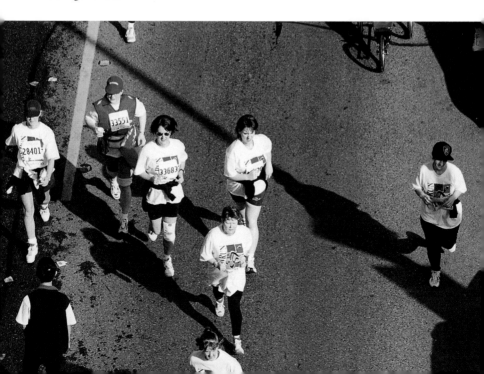

# Race Gear Checklist

**Shoes**
The best shoes to race in are the ones in which you trained. Some folks like racing flats for shorter races, but with improved shoe technology making high-quality lightweight trainers available, most opt for their training shoes.

**Shorts**
There are some great technical fabrics that will keep you dry and chafe-free in a variety of conditions.

**Shirt**
Pick one that gives you both comfort and sun and wind protection.

**Cap**
A breathable, lightweight cap that will help keep you cool and keep the sun's damaging rays off of you during the race is a good choice.

**Socks**
Choose a comfortable pair that you have used in training.

**Warm-up gear**
Take along some warm-up gear, top and bottoms. An old T-shirt you don't mind losing is a good choice.

**Garbage bag**
A large garbage bag makes a great disposable gym bag to take to the race. If it rains, you can put a hole in the bottom for some fast, simple raingear to keep you dry before the start.

**Vaseline**
Petroleum jelly will keep you from chafing.

| | |
|---|---|
| **Second skin** | **This product, or another, such as NuSkin, will save you the pain of chafing or cover a training blister.** |
| **Race number** | **Make sure you have it and make sure you pin it on the singlet or shirt that you will be wearing in the race. Take a few extra pins.** |
| **Water bottle** | **Most good races will have adequate water along the course. If you're unsure of the frequency of the water stations, wear a torso pack to take your own water with you.** |
| **Timing chip** | **The new timing systems sometimes sell individual timing chips to racers. If you have one of these, be sure to take it with you.** |

# Race Day

## Morning of the Race

Set your alarm for about 2 hours before the race to give yourself time to get up, prepare your gear and arrive at the race site 45 minutes before the start. Allow yourself enough time to park, find the start, visit the washroom one last time and do a light, easy run to warm up your muscles so you will not have to start cold.

One of the most common questions I get asked is, *What should I eat on race morning?* It's tough to find an answer that will work for everyone, but here is the one that works for me and a lot of folks that have asked in the past: a large glass of water, 10 ounces (284 ml) of apple juice and a package of instant oatmeal. Instant oatmeal is a great race-morning meal: it is easy to make in a hotel room; it is a filling, warm meal that leaves you satisfied; and it does not upset your stomach.

I like a cup of coffee in the morning, so I make sure I have an extra glass of water to offset the diuretic effects of the caffeine. You are still trying to keep

CH. 18

yourself hydrated, so during the entire morning before the race, you should try to drink 4 to 6 ounces (115 to 170 ml) of water every 30 minutes.

A warm shower will help warm up and loosen your muscles. After your shower, rub some petroleum jelly on your underarms and on your thighs between your legs to prevent chafing. Men should also put some on their nipples; women along their bra line. The extra exertion of the race causes you to sweat more than normal, and as the sweat evaporates it leaves behind salt, which is the culprit that causes chafing.

Get dressed and do a final check to be sure you have your race number on, and then put on your warm-up gear. If you have some extra time, do one last visualization to keep all your thoughts positive. Take any negative thoughts and turn them into positive affirmations.

You are now ready to leave for the race.

## Racing Tips

Whether you're a first-time fun runner or a seasoned road racer, the most important thing to remember is to stay relaxed. If you go down to your local track, you will hear the coach holler to the athletes, *Relax! Stay smooth! Push*

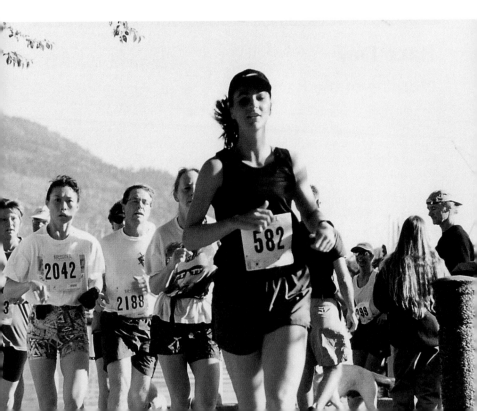

*hard!* It almost sounds like a contradiction, but both the coaches and the athletes will tell you that the more they relax, the easier it is for them to achieve their optimum performance. Stay relaxed, keep things in perspective and use common sense. Control the things you can control, and for other things remember you can run again on a new day.

- Do your warm-up on the last mile of the race to set the image of the finish area in your mind.

- Keep your pace within your training. Remember that even pace is not even effort: even pace requires you to hold back in the early stages and push harder in the last section. Break the race into thirds: the first third should seem very easy; the middle third should seem just right; the last third should require you to work hard to maintain the pace. Do this and you will run an even pace.

- Drink at the water stations. Walking through the water station will allow you to get more water into your body. If you get in a rush, you might miss and hit the guy running beside you or end up getting the water up your nose.

- Watch your stride: shorten your stride on the uphills; let gravity carry you down the hills as you maintain your stride. If you start to tire, focus in on your stride. Think of yourself running on hot coals to keep your leg turnover fast.

- Everyone goes through a negative period in their thinking during a race. Have a positive thought game plan to combat negativity. I like to think of having a fishing rod that I use to reel in the runner ahead of me. It gets you into the right brain mode, and as long as you don't take yourself too seriously, it also gets you to laugh.

- Remember that the race officials have measured the race on the tangents (the shortest distance between each corner), so run that line. Runners can be like cattle: we have a tendency to blindly follow the runner in front of us and occasionally we will be running farther as a result.

- Your primary goal should be to finish in a smiling, upright position. There are usually cameras in the finish area, so looking good is the best choice at this point, but don't finish with a sprint. Stay relaxed and finish with a strong form.

- As you finish, be sure to keep walking around to cool down. Drink liquids and eat some high-carbohydrate foods as soon as possible.

CH. 18

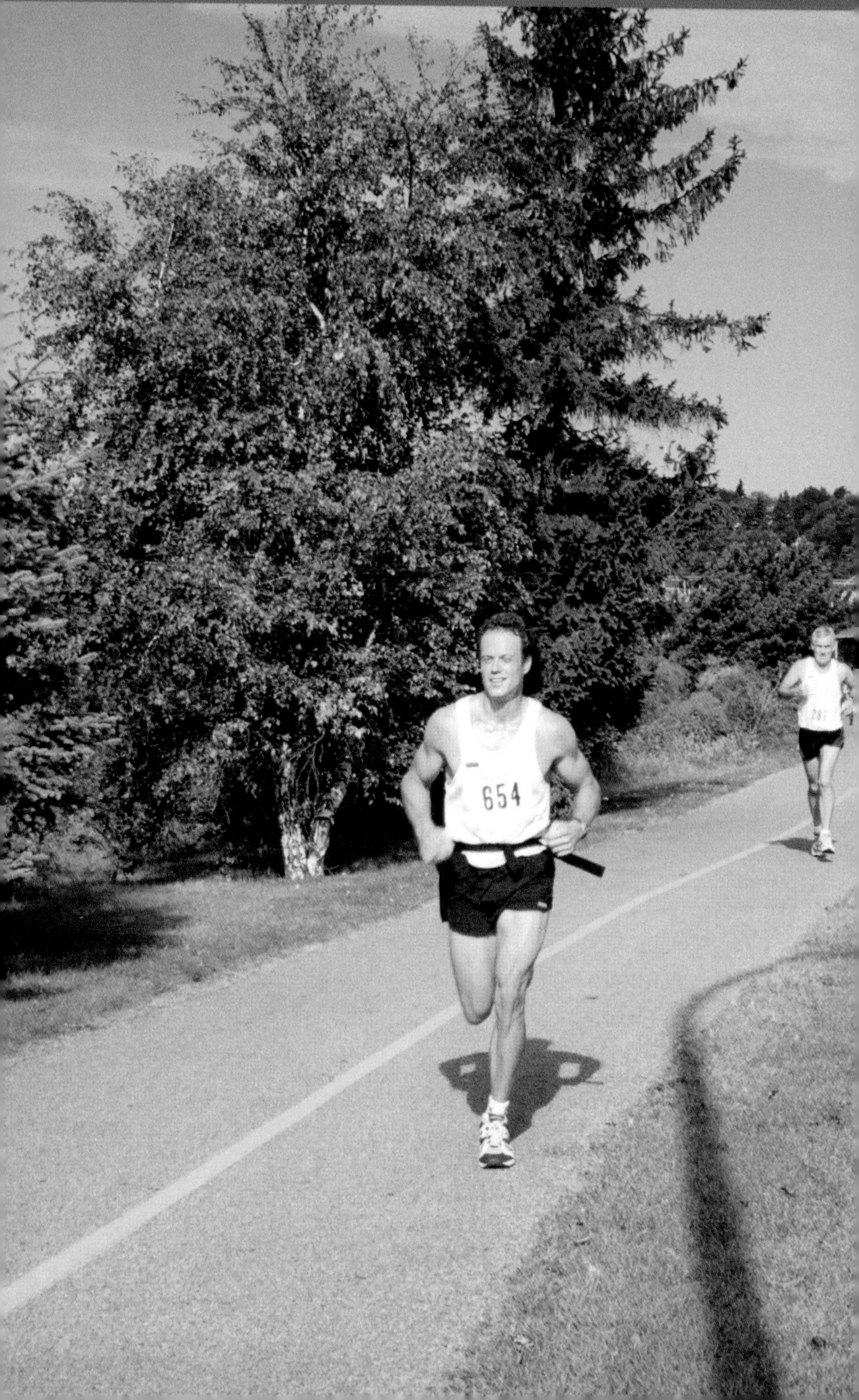
654

## Eating and Drinking for a Race

- Drink 6 ounces (170 ml) of water every hour during the day before the race.

- Drink 4 to 6 ounces (115 to 170 ml) of water every 30 minutes during the morning of the race.

- Caffeine and alcohol will dehydrate you.

- The early water stops are the most important.

- Stay with foods and drinks that have worked before. Don't try anything new for the race.

- Your last big meal should be lunch on the day before.

- Don't eat too much the night before.

- Carbohydrate drinks are easier to digest than solid food.

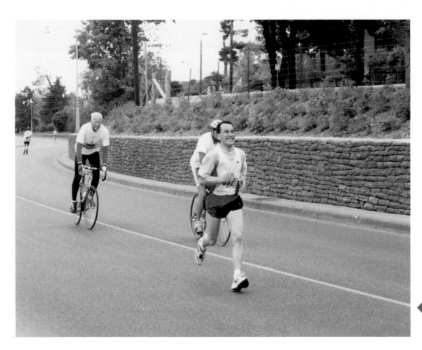

CH. 18

## Race Form Clarifications

**Flat and fast: boring run in the parking lot of a shopping centre.**

**Undulating: killer hills.**

**High-quality T-shirt: you hope it won't shrink.**

**Scenic course: you run past a shopping centre.**

**Awards ceremony: speechmaking that sometimes take longer than the race itself.**

**Breaking wind: taking the lead into a headwind when working together as a group.**

**Tangent: a legal running short cut.**

**Recovery time: the amount of time it takes to forget how bad racing felt so you're ready to do another one.**

**Well-hydrated: you cannot leave the area of the wash-rooms.**

# The Last 100 Metres

The highlight of the race comes in the last 100 metres. Much has been written about the various stages of a race, in particular the marathon. The famous "wall" has entertained many readers, but the true joy and rewards usually come in the final 100 metres or so of any race.

I have seen many a self-professed big tough runner brought to tears of joy as they run the final 100 metres. Watch the finish of a marathon, you will see the joy of success mixed with the tears and toil of hard work that has brought the runner to the finish line.

The real elation comes from the fact that each runner has pushed and paced themselves though the various difficult stages of the race. They have gone through the high and low points of the race and now can savour the sweet smell of the successful finish. Every runner that crosses the finish line knows that they have achieved success and are all winners in life as well as in the race.

CH. 18

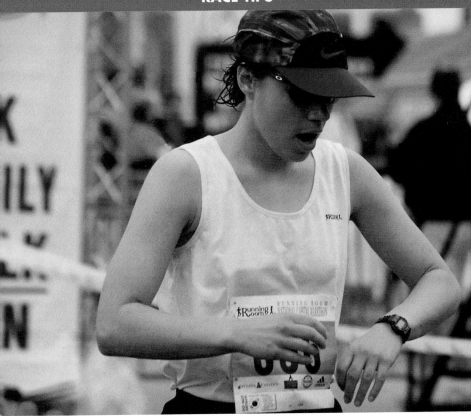

Runners learn that during the race they need to focus in on the goals of the day to get through the low points of the race. Experience teaches us that during each race, everyone goes through some low points where they ask, Why am I in this race? We think: I like running but I don't like racing. It hurts. Why don't I just quit? Who will know? I'm too old for this, people are asking why is that runner even in the race? I could just drop out and never enter a race again, no one would notice. I could take the bus back and even stop for a muffin and cold juice. I'm too old, I'm too fat ....

We have all heard that negative side of our brain nagging away at us during these times. Well, that's when it's important for you to take control of the situation and get the old positive brain—the "I feel great about everything" side—kick-started to take control of things.

The best way is to think about something that requires your creative brain. A technique you can use is to run the final 100 metres of the race during the warm-up. That way, when you're running in the race and are at a point where you're struggling, focus on that final 100 metres, or think of the final 100 metres of a previous race. Visualize the race finish banner, the crowd cheering you on and the race announcer's voice. See yourself finishing in control with powerful strides. You are strong; you are fit; your breathing is in control; you are in control. Feel the elation of the finish and savour the moment for future training runs and races. The final 100 metres is the self-motivational start of your next goal.

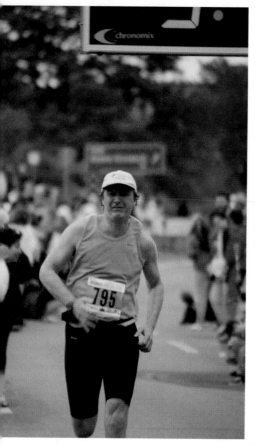

# After the Race

The time immediately after a race is a great time to get motivated to train again. Change into some clean, dry clothes and savour the electric feeling that comes after a run. Enjoy the company of the other runners.

Try to keep moving around after the race. It will help flush your muscles of any waste products that can leave you sore. In the evening, a warm bath will help you gently stretch any soreness in your muscles. If you are visiting a new city, the post-race afternoon is a great time to do some touring and model your new race T-shirt. You have special bragging rights for the balance of the day. You did it.

The day after the race is a good day to take off to allow your leg muscles to recover from the hard effort. You can swim or bike, if you want, because those activities will help loosen up your legs. I find that a swim after a race or hard training day is like a massage. Depending on the distance and your recovery, you may find that running only every other day during the week after a hard race will help the recovery of tired legs.

Often, after a race in which everything has gone well, you will be left with a new sense of motivation and confidence that will get you right back to your training with some new vigour and enthusiasm.

CH. 18

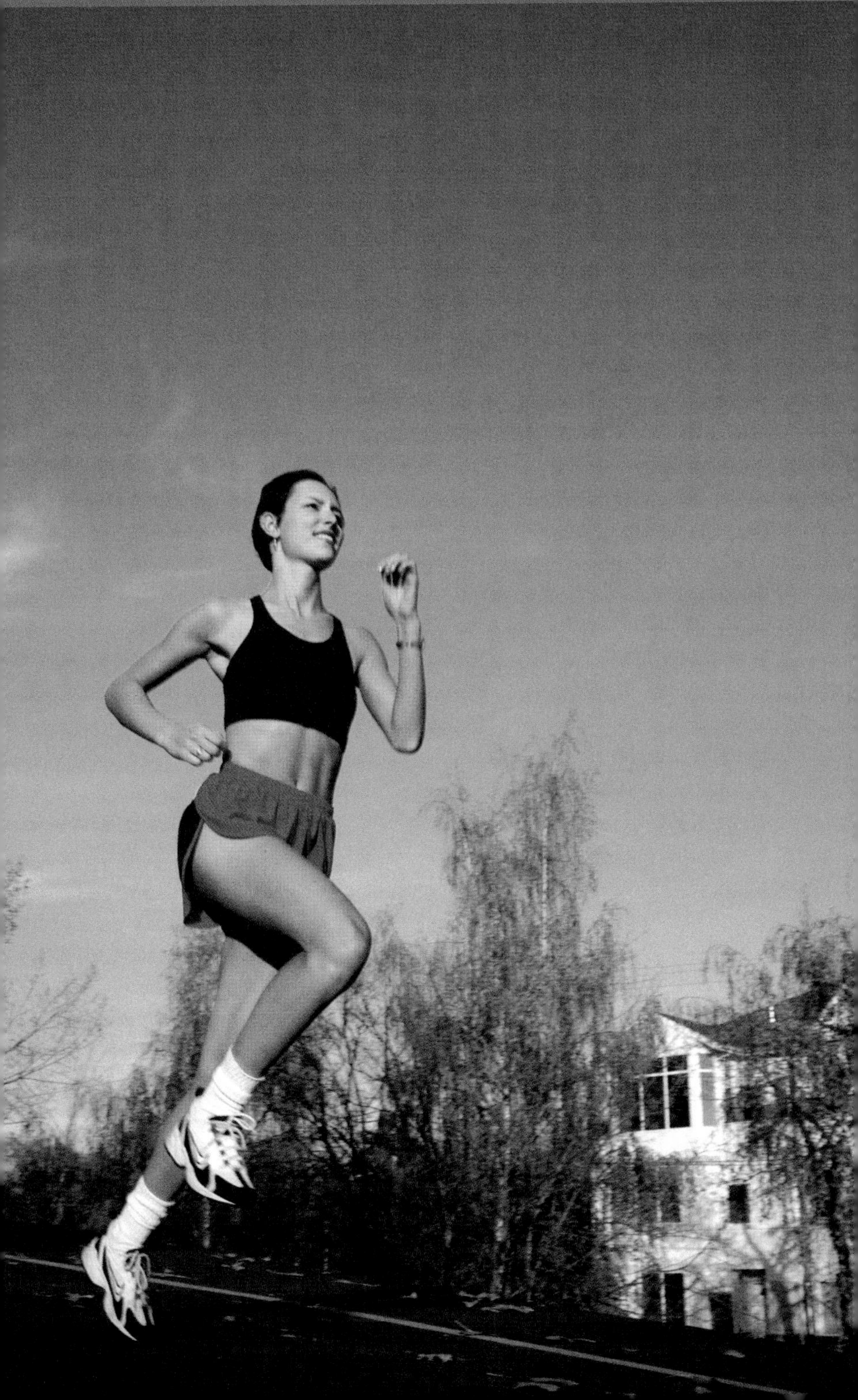

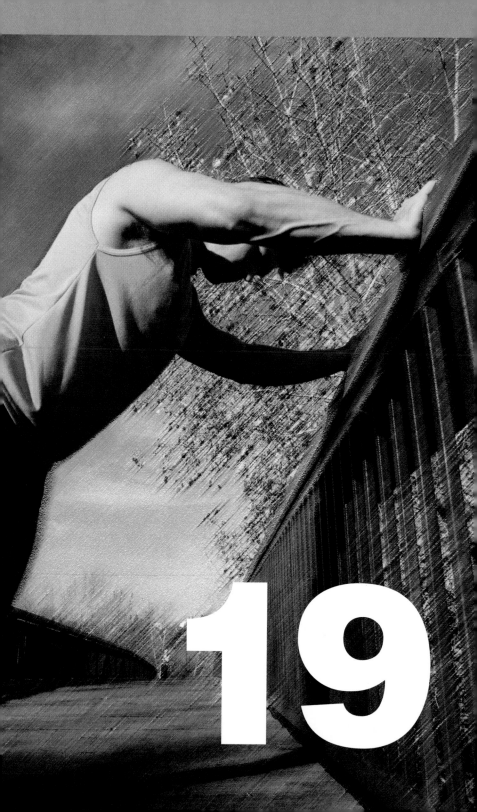

**19**

# Mental Preparation

What makes elite athletes perform to gold medal standards? What is it that motives them to perform better than their peers? If you study their training programs, most are similar to those used by folks they are competing with. Ask most coaches and they will quickly tell you that their primary job is to mentally prepare the athlete for competition.

Not every athlete can have the benefit of an individual coach, but the advice in this chapter can give you a tremendous advantage over your individual competitors. It will increase your personal performance, whether your target is to beat the last time you ran a particular distance or if you are about to run a challenging new distance.

## Relaxation

To start with, get yourself in a comfortable space. It could be sitting in a big soft chair, lying on your hotel bed or lying on the floor. The key is to spend a few moments just getting comfortable and relaxed. Put on some music that relaxes you. Take your mind off your worries or stress. Close your eyes and listen to the music, to the individual instruments, notes and sounds that make up the musical selection. Focus on the music, thinking only of the music and your body lying in the comfortable position.

Think of your body as a fine-tuned musical instrument ready to perform. Think back to all the positive training experiences your have had in preparation for the event. Think only positive thoughts. Relax and listen to your breathing. Breathe in, hold, breathe out. Feel the air filling your lungs that have trained and are now ready for the challenge of the day. Feel your heart rate lowering as you listen to the sound of your own breathing. Turn down the music and focus in on your healthy, fit body.

Start with the top of your head. Relax. Let the stress of the day leave your mind. Breathe in, hold, breathe out. Feel your forehead relax and the frown line between your eyes relax and disappear. Your eyelids are heavy and relaxed. Feel your jaw grow heavy with the relaxation. Open your mouth in a relaxed yawn. Roll your neck to relax the muscles of the neck and shoulders. If you are right-handed, start to concentrate on the right side of your body. Feel it getting heavy and relaxed. If you are left-handed, concentrate on the left side of the body.

Feel your shoulders heavy with the relaxed, peaceful feeling. Think of your body: strong, fit and ready. Your shoulders are now relaxed. Breathe in, hold, breathe out. Feel the air filling your lungs. Feel your abdominal muscles relaxing as you breathe out. Your back is relaxed; you feel the tenseness slowly leave the muscles, leaving them heavy and relaxed. Feel your hips heavy against the floor. Relax. Breathe in, hold, breathe out.

Feel your hamstrings and quadriceps, strong and ready from the months of training, now relaxed and rested. Feel the calf muscles that give you that special leveraged drive in your running, now relaxed and still. Breathe in, hold, breathe out. Roll your ankles and feel the relaxation all through your feet—the feet that are ready to carry you to your goal. Breathe in, hold, breathe out.

Listen to the stillness. Breathe in, hold, breathe out. There is no sound, just the rhythmic breathing of your relaxed body as your mind focuses on your visualization of the race.

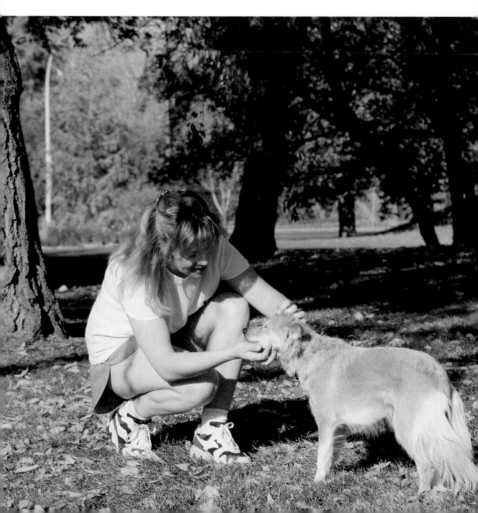

# 10-K Visualization

It is the morning of the race. You see yourself walking to the start area where runners have started to gather. You see the activity throughout the area: the race pick-up area with runners standing in line for their kits; some runners are stretching; some are jogging lightly; others are doing short wind sprints to ready themselves for the competition. You are quiet as you approach. You hear the sound of the race announcer calling for people to pick up their kits in time for the start. You hear the sound of other runners laughing and talking. You sense the excitement in the air, mixed with the early sunrise and the smell of athletic rub. The smell of fresh coffee in the volunteer area reminds you that it is time for you to rise to the occasion.

You know you are ready. You have done your training. You repeat your power words: you are strong, you are in control, you are fit, you feel good.

You see yourself talking to some running buddies as you give your running gear a final check. You smile to yourself as you hear some of the familiar pre-race comments: "I'm only doing this as a training run." "My knee is sore. I think I'll just jog this one." "Haven't been training much—that old Achilles has been acting up." "I had planned on racing this but I think I'll just take it easy, the hip's a little sore." You smile once again because you know all of the minor aches and pains disappear as soon as the start gun goes off.

You take that last drink of water as you head to the start line to join the group of people already in position. Runners are now all standing, nervously awaiting the start. Some are quiet; some are laughing nervously; others are staring and holding their wrists, ready to start their watches. All are awaiting the signal to start.

The announcer gives out some last-minute instructions and counts down to the start. The gun goes off and you start running.

You have seeded yourself well, but there is still a little bumping as the occasional runner brushes by you. You get around a couple of runners who are still walking and talking as you breeze by them. You gradually pick up the pace and then settle into your own rhythm. You are fluid and strong … you feel good. It is a good day as the warmth of the sun warms your shoulders and a light breeze cools your forehead.

You pass the 1-mile mark and you hear the time being called. You're right on target. You now concentrate on keeping the pace. You remember that the first third of the race you should be holding back; the middle third will feel just right; you will have to work hard in the final third. The key is an even pace—not even effort, but a modified effort throughout the race. You know your training has taught you the importance of holding back at the start and how to

CH. 19

time the extra effort that is needed in the latter stages of the race. You remember practising this in your training.

As you continue past the 1-mile mark you are now running in a group of several other runners. The occasional runner passes the group and the group passes a small group of three runners talking and joking to one another that they started a little fast. You know you started in control and are right on target. More importantly you feel great. You're strong—you have done the training.

You pass the 2-mile mark and you do your system check: your breathing is relaxed and controlled, your form is strong, your leg turnover is fast and fluid. You are looking and feeling good. You have settled into a comfortable, rhythmic pace. This is the part of the race that feels good; the pace seems easy as you flow along with the group of runners.

You spot the 5-km mark—halfway there and you are feeling strong and in control. As you pass the 5-km mark, you notice you are pulling away from some of the runners. Your group is growing smaller. You hold your pace, check your time. You are right on target as you enter the second half of the race. You check your form in your shadow on the road and focus on your stride, which is strong. Your breathing is even and you say to yourself: *I am strong, I am in control, I am fit, I am focused, I feel good, I am fast.*

## Positive Self-suggestions

- **I am in control of my own thinking, my own focus, my own life.**

- **I control my own thoughts and emotions and direct the whole pattern of my performance, health and life.**

- **I am fully capable of achieving the goals I set for my self today. They are within my control.**

- **I learn from problems, or setbacks, and through them I see room for improvement and opportunities for personal growth.**

- **Every day in some way I am better, wiser, more adaptable, more focused, more confident, more in control.**

You come up on the 8-km mark, the point where most runners start to question why they are racing: *Why not just run? Who needs to race when you can just run for fun?* You laugh and smile as you recognize the familiar negative thoughts that come at this part of the race. You know you are in control and focus in on your form. Listen to your footsteps, light on the ground. You say to yourself, *Hang in there, you're looking good.* Concentrate on shortening your stride and increasing your leg turnover. *I feel better already. I can do it.*

One mile to go and you are feeling strong. You know you are going to hit your target. You're fatigued but you know you can dig a little deeper and achieve that goal. Your stride improves as you can hear the noise of the finish line. You push yourself, increasing the tempo. You pass one, then two more runners. You're fit. You feel your breathing becoming laboured. Breathe in, fill your lungs with energy, breathe out, feel the negative feeling leave, feel the strong sense of well-being.

Adrenaline kicks in as you hear and see the finish line. Your stride opens up as you pass a couple of runners accelerating towards the finish line. Your form is fluid and strong. You knew you could do it! Your leg turnover increases rapidly. It is like you are running on hot coals. Your pace continues to quicken. You pass two more runners as you near the finish line. The announcer calls out your name and time. You have done it—you hit your target. You slow to a walk in the finish area, your hands on your hips as you thank your body for the effort. You give thanks to the good health and hard training that have enabled you to complete the race and be rewarded with this euphoric sense of well-being and accomplishment.

You know that with the proper physical training and the right mental preparation, you can achieve any goal you set for yourself; that reality is a creation of the way we see ourselves in our own minds.

# Marathon Visualization

The day you have been looking for has finally arrived. After months of self-discipline and hard training, it is the morning of the marathon. You are rested and well hydrated. You are making you way to the start/finish area. You know you are ready. You are in the midst of other runners, some talking, some silent and pensive, others laughing and joking. You can feel and sense the excitement in the area. There is a mixture of nervous adrenaline and anticipation as the sun begins to brighten and warm the area. The grass is damp with the morning dew as you set you sports bag down and pull off your sweat top to start you pre-race preparation. The music and noise is interrupted with the announcer calling out last-minute instructions to the runners. You take your final drink of water while zipping up your bag to turn it over to the check-in folks.

CH. 19

You make your way into the crowd to seed yourself with other runners who will be running about the same pace as you plan to run. Suddenly, it is quiet for a moment as you hear the announcer call, "Five … Four … Three … Two … One …."

The gun sounds and you are off. At first, it is more of a shuffle than a run as laughter and noise again fill the air. You hear a mixture of race chatter both from the runners and the people lining the course at the start.

Slowly, the crowd around you starts to open up and you start to find that familiar stride. Your breathing is now relaxed and you feel comfortable as you make the first turn on the course and head down the long straight-away. You are passed by a couple of runners who are joking with one another as they find their own pace. Just as you pass a small pack of five or six runners you realize you are already at the 1-mile mark. Are you right on target, did you start a little fast, or did the crowd slow you? Either way, this is only a benchmark to adjust your pace. You are feeling good. You think back to the months of training, some of it done with the group but a good portion done on your own. You know that those runs will pay big dividends to you today in your marathon.

At the 2-mile mark you do your first systems check. Are you relaxed? Is your breathing relaxed and are you taking deep, full breaths? Is your chest out, hips forward? Have you started to sweat yet? Is your head straight, eyes up the road, spotting a runner ahead? Arms relaxed and in tune with the rhythm of your running, you feel the confident push off each ankle. You feel and look good. This is your day and you are going to do your best.

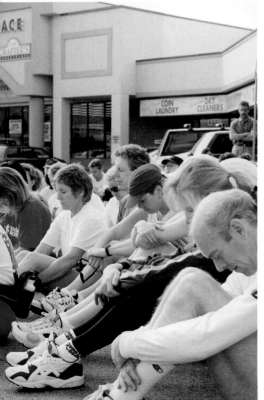

At the 5-mile mark you come out of a park area and start up the hill. You shorten your stride slightly, just like you did in all of those hill repeat sessions. This is a piece of cake; you did 10 to 12 hill repeats on a lot steeper hills than this. You continue with even effort as you head up the hill, passing a runner who appears to be struggling, while you are smooth and fluid. As you near the top of the hill you automatically run over the crest, just like in your training. You are now back on a flat stretch and regain the old familiar rhythm. You think back to those long runs with your training buddies. This is just another long run. Stay relaxed and enjoy the sights and sounds.

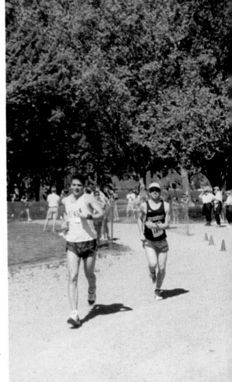

As you pass through a water station, there are people dressed in costumes cheering you on. Whoever talked about the loneliness of the long-distance runner? This is fun, this is life! You are getting to experience something less than one-tenth of 1 percent of the population ever has the good health and fitness to accomplish: you are running your marathon.

As you pass the halfway mark, you remember your power words: *I am strong; I am in control; I feel good.* As you say them to yourself, you feel the power boost they give you, both mentally and physically, as your legs respond to the familiar, comforting words.

You are passing through an older part of the city now filled with character, history and friendly enthusiastic crowds of people calling words of encouragement to you. Someone hands you a cup of water and you drink it in, feeling the cool, clear water on your throat. It is refreshing. It is refilling not only your liquids but you can feel the confidence build as you start to realize you are way past halfway. You repeat your power words. You are strong. You are in control. You are a strong and powerful athlete, well trained and prepared. You feel good, your body and mind are in rhythm with each other. As you repeat your power words, you feel them fill you with confidence and strength. You can do this. You have taken the challenge and you will succeed.

As you pass the 20-mile mark, you start down a hill. You feel like you're not doing this by yourself as that old training buddy gravity gives you a little push on the downhill section. You know that this is the tough part of the race, but you also know that you are ready. You think back to some of the long runs when you felt tired and you were not always sure you would make it, but you did, and after completing them you felt great.

CH. 19

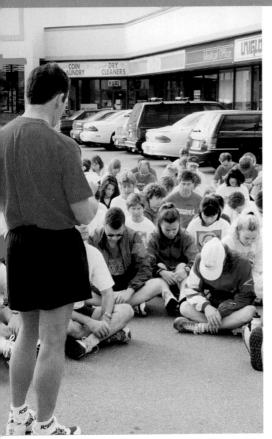

You think back to some of the games you played with yourself on the long runs, like the one with the fishing rod where you cast out the line to the runner ahead of you and then ever so gradually started to reel him in. You laugh to yourself as you focus in on the runners ahead and slowly, ever so slowly, you start to gain on them.

You now have less than 3 miles to go. You are strong and feeling confident as you start to pass runners. Some of them passed you earlier but you chose to let them go. They are now walking. You pass them and pick up the pace as you realize this is your day, your race and you prepared well and are now ready. You think for a moment of the finish area …. Just then you hear the announcer's voice and the cheers of the crowd in the finish area. A feeling of well-being and joy comes over you as you instinctively start to surge ahead and pass a couple of more runners who appear to be struggling. You are alone and running strong; you are really in control.

You begin to say your power words one last time: *I am strong. I am in control. I am fit and a powerful runner. I am a strong runner. I am fast and fluid.*

As you cross over the final bridge and start towards the finish line, you can hear the cheering of the crowd, the screaming of the cheerleaders, the race announcer calling your name ….

You cross the line and someone asks you if you are OK. You smile, unable to speak. You feel that special euphoric feeling that is somewhere between joy and the pain of the moment. With your hands on your hips, you walk towards the refreshment area, medal around your neck. You did it! You ran a marathon and you know that the confidence you now have will help in accomplishing any challenge you set for yourself. Even with all of life's speed bumps and challenges, you will achieve success because of the confidence that today has brought to you. You are a marathon runner! You know that any time you set a goal, train and work hard towards it, and dream of it, you will eventually achieve it in reality.

## Last Words

Take a moment now to think of your breathing and gradually come back to the time and place of the moment. Think of the response of all of the Olympians when asked what they thought was their greatest asset: they all said it was mental toughness and confidence. For all of us, we should practise this mental training often and in concert with our physical training.

### Positive Self-talk

- **I am in control of my own life.**

- **I can achieve any intelligent goal I set for myself.**

- **I believe in myself and the people around me.**

- **I treat every day as a new challenge to improve myself in some way.**

CH. 19

# Appendix: Marathon Pace Charts

## Kilometre Schedule

| Km Pace | 1 Mile | 5 km | 10 km | 15 km | 20 km |
|---------|--------|------|-------|-------|-------|
| 0:02:55 | 0:04:42 | 0:14:35 | 0:29:10 | 0:43:45 | 0:58:20 |
| 0:03:00 | 0:04:50 | 0:15:00 | 0:30:00 | 0:45:00 | 1:00:00 |
| 0:03:05 | 0:04:58 | 0:15:25 | 0:30:50 | 0:46:15 | 1:01:40 |
| 0:03:10 | 0:05:06 | 0:15:50 | 0:31:40 | 0:47:30 | 1:03:20 |
| 0:03:15 | 0:05:14 | 0:16:15 | 0:32:30 | 0:48:45 | 1:05:00 |
| 0:03:20 | 0:05:22 | 0:16:40 | 0:33:20 | 0:50:00 | 1:06:40 |
| 0:03:25 | 0:05:30 | 0:17:05 | 0:34:10 | 0:51:15 | 1:08:20 |
| 0:03:30 | 0:05:38 | 0:17:30 | 0:35:00 | 0:52:30 | 1:10:00 |
| 0:03:35 | 0:05:46 | 0:17:55 | 0:35:50 | 0:53:45 | 1:11:00 |
| 0:03:40 | 0:05:54 | 0:18:20 | 0:36:40 | 0:55:00 | 1:13:20 |
| 0:03:45 | 0:06:02 | 0:18:45 | 0:37:30 | 0:56:15 | 1:15:00 |
| 0:03:50 | 0:06:10 | 0:19:10 | 0:38:20 | 0:57:30 | 1:16:40 |
| 0:03:55 | 0:06:18 | 0:19:35 | 0:39:10 | 0:58:45 | 1:18:20 |
| 0:04:00 | 0:06:26 | 0:20:00 | 0:40:00 | 1:00:00 | 1:20:00 |
| 0:04:05 | 0:06:34 | 0:20:25 | 0:40:50 | 1:01:15 | 1:21:40 |
| 0:04:10 | 0:06:42 | 0:20:50 | 0:41:40 | 1:02:30 | 1:23:20 |
| 0:04:15 | 0:06:50 | 0:21:15 | 0:42:30 | 1:03:45 | 1:25:00 |
| 0:04:20 | 0:06:58 | 0:21:40 | 0:43:20 | 1:05:00 | 1:26:40 |
| 0:04:25 | 0:07:06 | 0:22:05 | 0:44:10 | 1:06:15 | 1:28:20 |
| 0:04:30 | 0:07:14 | 0:22:30 | 0:45:00 | 1:07:30 | 1:30:00 |
| 0:04:35 | 0:07:23 | 0:22:55 | 0:45:50 | 1:08:45 | 1:31:40 |
| 0:04:40 | 0:07:31 | 0:23:20 | 0:46:40 | 1:10:00 | 1:33:20 |
| 0:04:45 | 0:07:39 | 0:23:45 | 0:47:30 | 1:11:15 | 1:35:00 |
| 0:04:50 | 0:07:47 | 0:24:10 | 0:48:20 | 1:12:30 | 1:36:40 |
| 0:04:55 | 0:07:55 | 0:24:35 | 0:49:10 | 1:13:45 | 1:38:20 |
| 0:05:00 | 0:08:03 | 0:25:00 | 0:50:00 | 1:15:00 | 1:40:00 |
| 0:05:05 | 0:08:11 | 0:25:25 | 0:50:50 | 1:16:15 | 1:41:40 |
| 0:05:10 | 0:08:19 | 0:25:50 | 0:51:40 | 1:17:30 | 1:43:20 |

| Halfway (21.1 km) | 25 km | 30 km | 35 km | 40 km | Marathon (42.2 km) |
|---|---|---|---|---|---|
| 1:01:32 | 1:12:55 | 1:27:30 | 1:42:05 | 1:56:40 | 2:03:04 |
| 1:03:17 | 1:15:00 | 1:30:00 | 1:45:00 | 2:00:00 | 2:06:35 |
| 1:05:03 | 1:17:05 | 1:32:30 | 1:47:55 | 2:03:20 | 2:10:06 |
| 1:06:48 | 1:19:10 | 1:35:00 | 1:50:50 | 2:06:40 | 2:13:37 |
| 1:08:34 | 1:21:15 | 1:37:30 | 1:53:45 | 2:10:00 | 2:17:08 |
| 1:10:19 | 1:23:20 | 1:40:00 | 1:56:40 | 2:13:20 | 2:20:39 |
| 1:12:05 | 1:25:25 | 1:42:30 | 1:59:35 | 2:16:40 | 2:24:10 |
| 1:13:50 | 1:27:30 | 1:45:00 | 2:02:30 | 2:20:00 | 2:27:41 |
| 1:15:35 | 1:29:35 | 1:47:30 | 2:05:25 | 2:23:20 | 2:31:12 |
| 1:17:21 | 1:31:40 | 1:50:00 | 2:08:20 | 2:26:40 | 2:34:43 |
| 1:19:06 | 1:33:45 | 1:52:30 | 2:11:15 | 2:30:00 | 2:38:14 |
| 1:20:52 | 1:35:50 | 1:55:00 | 2:14:10 | 2:33:20 | 2:41:45 |
| 1:22:37 | 1:37:55 | 1:57:30 | 2:17:05 | 2:36:40 | 2:45:16 |
| 1:24:23 | 1:40:00 | 2:00:00 | 2:20:00 | 2:40:00 | 2:48:47 |
| 1:26:08 | 1:42:05 | 2:02:30 | 2:22:55 | 2:43:20 | 2:52:18 |
| 1:27:54 | 1:44:10 | 2:05:00 | 2:25:50 | 2:46:40 | 2:55:49 |
| 1:29:39 | 1:46:15 | 2:07:30 | 2:28:45 | 2:50:00 | 2:59:20 |
| 1:31:25 | 1:48:20 | 2:10:00 | 2:31:40 | 2:53:20 | 3:02:51 |
| 1:33:10 | 1:50:25 | 2:12:30 | 2:34:35 | 2:56:40 | 3:06:22 |
| 1:34:56 | 1:52:30 | 2:15:00 | 2:37:30 | 3:00:00 | 3:09:53 |
| 1:36:41 | 1:54:35 | 2:17:30 | 2:40:25 | 3:03:20 | 3:13:24 |
| 1:38:27 | 1:56:40 | 2:20:00 | 2:43:20 | 3:06:40 | 3:16:55 |
| 1:40:12 | 1:58:45 | 2:22:30 | 2:46:15 | 3:10:00 | 3:20:26 |
| 1:41:58 | 2:00:50 | 2:25:00 | 2:49:10 | 3:13:20 | 3:23:57 |
| 1:43:43 | 2:02:55 | 2:27:30 | 2:52:05 | 3:16:40 | 3:27:28 |
| 1:45:29 | 2:05:00 | 2:30:00 | 2:55:00 | 3:20:00 | 3:30:59 |
| 1:47:14 | 2:07:05 | 2:32:30 | 2:57:55 | 3:23:20 | 3:34:29 |
| 1:49:00 | 2:09:10 | 2:35:00 | 3:00:50 | 3:26:40 | 3:38:00 |

# MARATHON PACE CHARTS

| Km Pace | 1 Mile | 5 km | 10 km | 15 km | 20 km |
|---------|--------|------|-------|-------|-------|
| 0:05:15 | 0:08:27 | 0:26:15 | 0:52:30 | 1:18:45 | 1:45:00 |
| 0:05:20 | 0:08:35 | 0:26:40 | 0:53:20 | 1:20:00 | 1:46:40 |
| 0:05:25 | 0:08:43 | 0:27:05 | 0:54:10 | 1:21:15 | 1:48:20 |
| 0:05:30 | 0:08:51 | 0:27:30 | 0:55:00 | 1:22:30 | 1:50:00 |
| 0:05:35 | 0:08:59 | 0:27:55 | 0:55:50 | 1:23:45 | 1:51:40 |
| 0:05:40 | 0:09:07 | 0:28:20 | 0:56:40 | 1:25:00 | 1:53:20 |
| 0:05:45 | 0:09:15 | 0:28:45 | 0:57:30 | 1:26:15 | 1:55:00 |
| 0:05:50 | 0:09:23 | 0:29:10 | 0:58:20 | 1:27:30 | 1:56:40 |
| 0:05:55 | 0:09:31 | 0:29:35 | 0:59:10 | 1:28:45 | 1:58:20 |
| 0:06:00 | 0:09:39 | 0:30:00 | 1:00:00 | 1:30:00 | 2:00:00 |
| 0:06:05 | 0:09:47 | 0:30:25 | 1:00:50 | 1:31:15 | 2:01:40 |
| 0:06:10 | 0:09:55 | 0:30:50 | 1:01:40 | 1:32:30 | 2:03:20 |
| 0:06:15 | 0:10:03 | 0:31:15 | 1:02:30 | 1:33:45 | 2:05:00 |

## Mile Schedule

| Mile Pace | 5 miles | 10 miles | Halfway (13.1 mi) | 15 miles | 20 miles |
|-----------|---------|----------|-------------------|----------|----------|
| 0:04:40 | 0:23:20 | 0:46:40 | 1:01:11 | 1:10:00 | 1:33:20 |
| 0:04:50 | 0:24:10 | 0:48:20 | 1:03:22 | 1:12:30 | 1:36:40 |
| 0:05:00 | 0:25:00 | 0:50:00 | 1:05:33 | 1:15:00 | 1:40:00 |
| 0:05:10 | 0:25:50 | 0:51:40 | 1:07:44 | 1:17:30 | 1:43:20 |
| 0:05:15 | 0:26:15 | 0:52:30 | 1:08:49 | 1:18:45 | 1:45:00 |
| 0:05:20 | 0:26:40 | 0:53:20 | 1:09:55 | 1:20:00 | 1:46:50 |
| 0:05:30 | 0:27:30 | 0:55:00 | 1:12:06 | 1:22:30 | 1:50:00 |
| 0:05:40 | 0:28:20 | 0:56:40 | 1:14:17 | 1:25:00 | 1:53:20 |
| 0:05:45 | 0:28:45 | 0:57:30 | 1:15:23 | 1:26:15 | 1:55:00 |
| 0:05:50 | 0:29:10 | 0:58:20 | 1:16:28 | 1:27:30 | 1:56:40 |
| 0:06:00 | 0:30:00 | 1:00:00 | 1:18:39 | 1:30:00 | 2:00:00 |
| 0:06:10 | 0:30:50 | 1:01:40 | 1:20:50 | 1:32:30 | 2:03:20 |

# MARATHON PACE CHARTS

| Halfway (21.1 km) | 25 km | 30 km | 35 km | 40 km | Marathon (42.2 km) |
|---|---|---|---|---|---|
| 1:50:45 | 2:11:15 | 2:37:30 | 3:03:45 | 3:30:00 | 3:41:31 |
| 1:52:30 | 2:13:20 | 2:40:00 | 3:06:40 | 3:33:20 | 3:45:02 |
| 1:54:16 | 2:15:50 | 2:42:30 | 3:09:35 | 3:36:40 | 3:48:33 |
| 1:56:01 | 2:17:30 | 2:45:00 | 3:12:30 | 3:40:00 | 3:52:04 |
| 1:57:47 | 2:19:35 | 2:47:30 | 3:15:25 | 3:43:20 | 3:55:35 |
| 1:59:32 | 2:21:40 | 2:50:00 | 3:18:20 | 3:46:40 | 3:59:06 |
| 2:01:18 | 2:23:45 | 2:52:30 | 3:21:15 | 3:50:00 | 4:02:37 |
| 2:03:03 | 2:25:50 | 2:55:00 | 3:24:10 | 3:53:20 | 4:06:08 |
| 2:04:49 | 2:27:55 | 2:57:30 | 3:27:05 | 3:56:40 | 4:09:39 |
| 2:06:34 | 2:30:00 | 3:00:00 | 3:30:00 | 4:00:00 | 4:13:10 |
| 2:08:20 | 2:32:05 | 3:02:30 | 3:32:55 | 4:03:20 | 4:16:41 |
| 2:10:05 | 2:34:10 | 3:05:00 | 3:35:50 | 4:06:40 | 4:20:12 |
| 2:11:51 | 2:36:15 | 3:07:30 | 3:38:45 | 4:10:00 | 4:23:43 |

| 25 miles | Marathon (26.2 mi) |
|---|---|
| 1:56:40 | 2:02:21 |
| 2:00:50 | 2:06:43 |
| 2:05:00 | 2:11:06 |
| 2:09:10 | 2:15:28 |
| 2:11:15 | 2:17:39 |
| 2:13:20 | 2:19:50 |
| 2:17:30 | 2:24:12 |
| 2:21:40 | 2:28:34 |
| 2:23:45 | 2:30:45 |
| 2:25:50 | 2:32:57 |
| 2:30:00 | 2:37:19 |
| 2:34:10 | 2:41:41 |

# MARATHON PACE CHARTS

| Mile Pace | 5 miles | 10 miles | Halfway (13.1 mi) | 15 miles | 20 miles |
|---|---|---|---|---|---|
| 0:06:15 | 0:31:15 | 1:02:30 | 1:21:56 | 1:33:45 | 2:05:00 |
| 0:06:20 | 0:31:40 | 1:03:20 | 1:23:02 | 1:35:00 | 2:06:40 |
| 0:06:30 | 0:32:30 | 1:05:00 | 1:25:13 | 1:37:30 | 2:10:00 |
| 0:06:40 | 0:33:20 | 1:06:40 | 1:27:24 | 1:40:00 | 2:13:20 |
| 0:06:45 | 0:33:45 | 1:07:30 | 1:28:29 | 1:41:15 | 2:15:00 |
| 0:06:50 | 0:34:10 | 1:08:20 | 1:29:35 | 1:42:30 | 2:16:40 |
| 0:07:00 | 0:35:00 | 1:10:00 | 1:31:46 | 1:45:00 | 2:20:00 |
| 0:07:10 | 0:35:50 | 1:11:40 | 1:33:57 | 1:47:30 | 2:23:20 |
| 0:07:15 | 0:36:15 | 1:12:30 | 1:35:03 | 1:48:45 | 2:25:00 |
| 0:07:20 | 0:36:40 | 1:13:20 | 1:36:08 | 1:50:00 | 2:26:40 |
| 0:07:30 | 0:37:30 | 1:15:00 | 1:38:19 | 1:52:30 | 2:30:00 |
| 0:07:40 | 0:38:20 | 1:16:40 | 1:40:30 | 1:55:00 | 2:33:20 |
| 0:07:45 | 0:38:45 | 1:17:30 | 1:41:36 | 1:56:15 | 2:35:00 |
| 0:07:50 | 0:39:10 | 1:18:20 | 1:42:41 | 1:57:30 | 2:36:40 |
| 0:08:00 | 0:40:00 | 1:20:00 | 1:44:53 | 2:00:00 | 2:40:00 |
| 0:08:10 | 0:40:50 | 1:21:40 | 1:47:04 | 2:02:30 | 2:43:20 |
| 0:08:15 | 0:41:15 | 1:22:30 | 1:48:09 | 2:03:45 | 2:45:00 |
| 0:08:20 | 0:41:40 | 1:23:20 | 1:49:15 | 2:05:00 | 2:46:40 |
| 0:08:30 | 0:42:30 | 1:25:00 | 1:51:26 | 2:07:30 | 2:50:00 |
| 0:08:40 | 0:43:20 | 1:26:40 | 1:53:37 | 2:10:00 | 2:53:20 |
| 0:08:45 | 0:43:45 | 1:27:30 | 1:54:42 | 2:11:15 | 2:55:00 |
| 0:08:50 | 0:44:10 | 1:28:20 | 1:55:48 | 2:12:30 | 2:56:40 |
| 0:09:00 | 0:45:00 | 1:30:00 | 1:57:59 | 2:15:00 | 3:00:00 |
| 0:09:10 | 0:45:50 | 1:31:40 | 2:00:10 | 2:17:30 | 3:03:20 |
| 0:09:15 | 0:46:15 | 1:32:30 | 2:01:16 | 2:18:45 | 3:05:00 |
| 0:09:20 | 0:46:40 | 1:33:20 | 2:02:21 | 2:20:00 | 3:06:40 |
| 0:09:30 | 0:47:30 | 1:35:00 | 2:04:32 | 2:22:30 | 3:10:00 |
| 0:09:40 | 0:48:20 | 1:36:40 | 2:06:43 | 2:25:00 | 3:13:20 |
| 0:09:45 | 0:48:45 | 1:37:30 | 2:07:49 | 2:26:15 | 3:15:00 |
| 0:09:50 | 0:49:10 | 01:38.2 | 2:08:55 | 2:27:30 | 3:16:40 |
| 0:10:00 | 0:50:00 | 1:40:00 | 2:11:06 | 2:30:00 | 3:20:00 |

# About the Author

John Stanton, once an overweight, out-of-shape food executive, underwent a total lifestyle change after running in a 3-km road race with his sons. The couch potato turned into an athlete and went on to run many marathons, road races and triathlons, including the Hawaiian Ironman and the Canadian Ironman. John founded a specialty running store that now has outlets across North America. Through his running clinics he has successfully coached tens of thousands of runners with the philosophy that anyone can run and that running should be fun. His unique programs have helped many individuals achieve extraordinary fitness goals through intelligent and innovative training techniques.

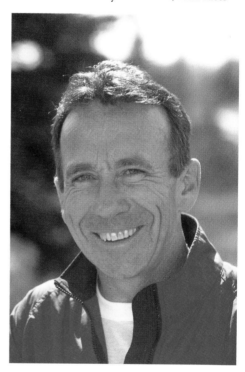

| 25 miles | Marathon (26.2 mi) |
|----------|--------------------|
| 2:36:15 | 2:43:52 |
| 2:38:20 | 2:46:03 |
| 2:42:30 | 2:50:25 |
| 2:46:40 | 2:54:48 |
| 2:48:45 | 2:56:59 |
| 2:50:50 | 2:59:10 |
| 2:55:00 | 3:03:32 |
| 2:59:10 | 3:07:54 |
| 3:01:15 | 3:10:05 |
| 3:03:20 | 3:12:16 |
| 3:07:30 | 3:16:38 |
| 3:11:40 | 3:21:01 |
| 3:13:45 | 3:23:12 |
| 3:15:50 | 3:25:23 |
| 3:20:00 | 3:29:45 |
| 3:24:10 | 3:34:07 |
| 3:26:15 | 3:36:18 |
| 3:28:20 | 3:38:29 |
| 3:32:30 | 3:42:52 |
| 3:36:40 | 3:47:14 |
| 3:38:45 | 3:49:25 |
| 3:40:50 | 3:51:36 |
| 3:45:00 | 3:55:58 |
| 3:49:10 | 4:00:20 |
| 3:51:15 | 4:02:31 |
| 3:53:20 | 4:04:42 |
| 3:57:30 | 4:09:05 |
| 4:01:40 | 4:13:27 |
| 4:03:45 | 4:15:38 |
| 4:05:50 | 4:17:49 |
| 4:10:00 | 4:22:11 |